Customize ME!

The First Ever Reader-Specific Publication

by: Scott Blaise

© 2016 by Scott Blaise. All rights reserved.

No part of this book may be reproduced in any written, electronic, recording or photocopying without written permission from the author, Scott Blaise, or the publisher, Blaise Publishing House, LLC.

Books may be purchased in quantity and/or special pricing by contacting the author by email; *questions@scottblaise.com*

Published by Blaise Publishing House, LLC - Princeton, NJ
Interior Design by: Scott Blaise
Cover Design by: Scott Blaise
Edited by: Julie Bruder
Creative Consultant: Chef, Jenna Dawson

ISBN-13: 9781660010721

Second Edition
Printed in the USA

This book is dedicated to my three daughters; Mia, Alaina and Grace.

In the loving memory of my grandparents...you are missed each & every day!

Julie - Thank you for all the support, encouragement and hard work! I could not have republished this work without you.

Preface

With the ever increasing need for diet, fitness and lifestyle solutions that work, I set out to create the first ever reader-specific publication. Based upon the ancient philosophies of Ayurveda, I'm bringing forth these timeless traditions in an easy to understand format, thus, successfully bridging the gap between a lifelong forgotten and the fast-paced modern times of today. By doing so, you'll learn a systematic process allowing you the chance to successfully incorporate the theories and principles of Ayurveda effortlessly into your life.

The premise of this work is based solely on the fact that each of us are unique, and what is healthy for me may not be in fact healthy for you. Taking this proclamation a step further, what may be healthy for you in the summer may be disturbing in the winter. You are truly unique. You don't merely dress different, sound different and look different, but rather you are unique. Every cell in your body is a unique energetic construction which makes what you see in the mirror every day. By understanding your true nature and how it interacts with the foods you consume, the area in which you reside, and how you conduct your daily activities, you will then soon come to understand and be able to easily apply what is forthcoming in the coming chapters of this book.

By explaining the concepts of the five universal elements, your specific body type (*dosha*), the six tastes and their interaction with the flow of Universal intelligence, you will gain a true understanding of how life is meant to be experienced. Once this has been established and properly understood, I will intertwine the Three Pillars of health with how we think and live in today's modern society. You will discover that even the most trivial things like consuming water has to be done in a specific manner according to your unwavering constitution (*dosha*).

Since the basis of this book was created upon the foundation that we all must know, understand and be able to successfully apply to our truest nature to every aspect of our lives, the recommendations forthcoming can be nothing other than generalized suggestions. My goal in writing this book is to provide you with definitive information and a system specific to you and your one-of-a-kind constitution, so that you will never need to fall victim again to the latest diet fad or scam. With that said, by following the instructions at the end of this work, you will have the opportunity to secure your very own customized version of this book. This version will include a full assessment of your body-type (*dosha*), its current state, as well as specific meal plans, exercise routines and your overall daily lifestyle. If for whatever reason this is not possible at this time for you, I hope the structure, suggestions and theories I provide within the many pages of this book will allow you enough guidance and information to make the proper and positive changes in your life. I am curious to see what would happen if together we created an epidemic of health?

Note From the Author:

There are many terms within the ancient Ayurvedic texts which have no English equivalent, such as the word ""*dosha*". I will do my best in defining each term so that you can understand best these timeless traditions. For each Sanskrit word found throughout this work, there will easily be designated in *italics*. In some instances, I will intertwine both the original Sanskrit term as well as its English equivalent. Also, there are many times where I will use the term "universe and/or universal". When I am using the term in a direct reference to God or the Mind of God, the word will be capitalized. If the term is used in a generalized connotation, it will be penned in lower case characters.

Table of Contents

Preface	4
Table of Contents	7
Introduction	8
The Five Elements	10
Understanding the Real You	21
The Taste of it	36
Digestion, Do You Get it?	53
Eat to Nourish, not to Diet!	67
Mind, The Psychosomatic Effect	80
Eat Your Medicine	99
The Three Pillars of Health	120
Ayurveda and the Mind	136
Pathology & Disease	155
Lifestyle & Routine	164
The Vata Daily Routine	171
The Pitta Daily Routine	185
The Kapha Daily Routine	196
An Ancient Medicine for Modern Times	211
True Beauty Lives Within Dinacharya	242
Summation	274

Introduction

> "Foolish the doctor who despises the knowledge acquired by the ancients"
>
> - **Hippocrates**

Do you believe you are unique? Do you understand what this means and how to apply it to every aspect of your life? If you're unsure how to answer the prior, then you need to keep reading with an open mind and with an open heart. If you do, and truly understand just how unique you are then congratulations and perhaps together we can spread the word and ultimately create balance, peace and harmony within us all.

I am attempting to do something that has never been successfully attempted before. I am going out on a limb; I am putting myself out there by creating this work for you, specifically for you! Sure, the person standing next to you on the subway, or your wife, son, granddaughter, and even the person from the gym who throws you the occasional glance might be holding a copy of this book. It is different, however, and their copy is just as unique as you. Despite the fact that it may look the same, feel the same, and it's inner workings is built upon the same premise as yours...it is different. You are different! Not the same kind of different that your crazy Uncle Bob acts at the annual family cookout, but unique down to the very last cell of your body. Until you uncover, understand, and truly wrap this around every aspect of your life then everything you do, eat and ever think is nothing other than a gamble. We have all been gambling, all of us, everywhere, and with something far more valuable than money...we have been gambling with our lives.

Built upon a foundation of something that was revealed more generations ago than I can possibly fathom, this publication will be created with you in mind. Together we will write this manuscript; we will uncover and discover together your true nature. And it will be these words that will fill the many pages of your customized version of "Customize ME!". Use it as a guide, for it will be your bible. It is not the "Bible," but rather it will be your scripture, for once your uniqueness was set forth pre-birth it has been unchanged, unwavering and absolute. Sure, the color of your hair changes, your weight fluctuates, everyone's does, but our true self has remained constant. So relax, take a deep breath, close your eyes, and let's create and author what will be the last diet book you'll ever need.

The Five Elements

"Man is the epitome of the universe. Within man, there is as much diversity as in the world outside. Similarly, the outside world is as diverse as human beings themselves."

— **Charaka, Ancient Ayurvedic Text**

मनुष्य ब्रह्मांड का प्रतीक है। आदमी के भीतर, बाहर की दुनिया में जितनी विविधता है। इसी प्रकार, बाहरी दुनिया भी उतनी ही विविधतापूर्ण है जितनी कि मनुष्य स्वयं

manushy brahmaand ka prateek hai. aadamee ke bheetar, baahar kee duniya mein jitanee vividhata hai. isee prakaar, baaharee duniya bhee utanee hee vividhataapoorn hai jitanee ki manushy svayan

Let's start to unveil your true nature by beginning to understand what makes you so unique and different. Is the old saying "less is more" so true that the basis of our entire material universe can be built upon only five things? In Ayurveda, or better yet, in Samkhya, creation takes a unique and metaphysical stand regarding creation. It is twofold: *prakriti* is considered the material cause of the world and God is the mental cause[1]. *Prakriti*, as understood in Vedanta, is the prime material energy of which all matter is composed[2]. In Ayurveda when dealing with your physical and mental body, it is looked upon as your God-given constitution. You see, in every theory, religion, or scientific

---

[1] "Samkhya - Wikipedia." https://en.wikipedia.org/wiki/Samkhya. Accessed 2 Jan. 2017.

[2] "Prakṛti - Wikipedia." https://en.wikipedia.org/wiki/Prak%E1%B9%9Bti. Accessed 2 Jan. 2017.

system in the world, they have to account for the occurrence of certain events - every event must and does have a particular cause. The delicate interplay between cause and effect is all-encompassing, and you and I are certainly no exception to the rule.

According to Samkhya, something which is nonexistent cannot come into existence, and something which exists, can never be considered nonexistent. So in a sense, creation or manifestation simply occurs from something that is hidden, rather than something that is nonexistent. This philosophy closely marries what the sciences of today are now confirming. Generation and regeneration, construction and deconstruction, and birth and rebirth, are the changes from one aspect of the same thing to another. In seeing that Samkhya regards the universe as consisting of two realities: consciousness *Purusha* and material realm *Prakriti*, I find it of utmost importance that we take a brief moment to understand these two aspects of creation. You will learn in later chapters its relationship to the health of your body and life.

When dealing with the causation of matter, the theory of Ayurveda is quite clear; the 5 universal elements *(panchamahabhutas)*, are the energetic factors underlying what we would refer to as our bodies and the material world in and around us. These five things are the same five elements that make up all and everything we've come to know and even those things which we cannot see or understand. They are the essential building blocks of all matter; living and non-living – organic and inorganic[3].

---

[3] "Pancha Bhoota - Wikipedia." https://en.wikipedia.org/wiki/Pancha_Bhoota. Accessed 4 Jan. 2017.

I have often been asked over the years since everything is made up of only five single elements, then how can there be such variance and uniqueness in the world? It is simple; it is as simple as the fact that even the minutest degree of difference between these elements causes these subtle differences. It is these subtleties that forms the tree in your yard and has shaped your dog into what you've grown to love and cherish. These elements are universal, absolute, never-ending, and work together in one common law. Understanding this law and how you interact with these elements will be one of the main principles of this book, as well as one of the most important aspects of your life. These universal elements work and exist on the gross and subtle levels, and it is only in their gross forms do we then experience physical matter. The subtler aspects of these elements work on the level of man's subconscious and unconscious state, as in regards to the dream state. They are the principles of density which applies to all that is manifest, both in the physical and in the mental realms. As you will learn later in this work, everything is constructed out of these five elements, and understanding that the differences you witness with the five senses of man are nothing other than variations of the same substance.

Now, don't you worry, you will not need to perform the same ancient rituals which were practiced 4,000 B.C. This is for me to ponder. It is my job to interpret the writings, works, and philosophies of these ancient Seers. It is your job to be forthcoming, determined, and truthful. If you do, and we work together, the state of your health will never again be the same. Now, I am not saying you'll never fall ill or never again come down with a case of the sniffles. This is part of being human. What I am referring to goes much deeper and is far more serious and complex than a mere head cold. Open your mind and your heart, if even for a moment, and allow something new to bless your life.

These elements, or energetic forces, are constant and forever changing and are moving rhythmically to the laws of the universe. You do not have to be the Enlightened One to understand this, as modern science has even confirmed solid matter is, in fact, constructed from subtle moving energy at the subatomic level. It is in this context which I refer to when I say space, air, fire, water, and earth. This energy, the stuff in and around us, has been called many names by many people over the centuries, but despite the many masks it wears, I believe we are all talking about and referring to the same thing. We have to be because if we weren't then the differences in which I've referred to thus far would be immeasurable and unfathomable to the point of non-existence.

As we discuss, understand, and begin to apply the nature of the five universal elements to your daily life, you must understand that they work together, in the order stated, and when they are out of balance, they'll do the same to create what some of us experience daily as a headache, diabetes, or even worse. All disease originates as an imbalance of these universal elements - whether mental or physical.

There is one word that will play a great importance in how well you will understand and are able to apply the principles of this book to your everyday life. It is not a difficult word, and though I cannot remember exactly when I first learned this word, I imagine it was somewhere during the early years of elementary school. The word to which I am referring is "quality." Not the same meaning as in "he does quality work," but rather an essential or distinctive characteristic, property, or attribute.

Ask yourself this, what are the "qualities" of the foods that I consume? What are the qualities of the environment in which I live, and what are the inherent qualities of my mind and my body? Once you begin to understand the true nature of these things, it will be only then where you will no longer find yourself suffering from a chronic disease. Chronic illnesses are so prevalent in our society today. The sad fact is that most of them can be avoided, or at least greatly reduced. Never again will you have to worry about your weight nor will you feel ashamed by your physical appearance to the point that even leaving your house is not an option. We will take a closer look at the five universal elements below, but first, let's learn and understand the 20 qualities according to Ayurveda.

The 20 Qualities of Everything

Hot	Cold
Sharp	Dull
Hard	Soft
Dry	Wet
Heavy	Light
Rough	Smooth

Slow	Quick
Oily	Brittle
Solid	Liquid
Dense	Subtle

The qualities listed above may seem like ordinary words, but once you're finished reading and fully comprehending this book, these words will take on a completely different meaning than the ones you've come to understand. Every quality has its polar opposite, and it is through the unique balance of these opposites that we can truly learn how to bring an unbalanced body back into its natural state. The good news is that the body wants to be in a balanced state; the universal laws of nature govern this natural selection. It is easy to cognize, however, that an excess or deficiency with any of the above qualities will lead to an imbalance, thus manifesting as what we know as "dis" – "ease." As an example, if your body is oily and wet, you would want to what…? The action and efficacy of opposites are not only easy to grasp and put into action, but it becomes a vital method when trying to support a healthy and balanced body throughout the year.

Not only do these qualities affect the body and mind itself, but they provide an easy understanding of the nature of the food. Something which possesses the quality of "heaviness," such as meat, will be hard to digest. Something that is "cold," like most dairy products, causes a cold and heavy feeling. If you're a person who has a slow or diminished digestion and has just learned heavy foods are more difficult to digest, it would then stand to reason you'd want to avoid consuming foods of a heavy nature, correct? Not following this ever-important philosophy will result in the creation and accumulation of undigested food stuff (*ama*), thus surely manifesting at one time or another as disease. The 5 universal elements are as follows:

1. Space or Ether
2. Air
3. Fire
4. Water
5. Earth

The important aspect to understand when referring to the elements above, is that I am not always referring to them in context that we have been taught and grown accustomed to understanding. Their energetic factors are what you need to concern yourself with more when I refer to "earth". Let's take a moment here and describe the nature of each element and how they affect what you witness in the mirror each day.

Space or Ether

The first element we will discuss (again, these are listed in a progressive manner - nothing can exist unless there is space for it to exist and become) is space. Space, or often referred to as ether, is wide-open vastness. It is immobile and does not move. The manifestation of the space element allows for the other four elements to come into being and works in conjunction with each other in a progressive manner. Ether is the something that occupies the areas where we sense nothing at all exists. Space permeates everything we see and everything which we cannot see, taste, smell and touch. The qualities of space are soft, light, subtle and abundant. The quality of space provides room and openness. Space facilitates sound and is non-resistant. Space is anything that is light, profuse, and ethereal. An example of the space element in an everyday food is popcorn. Space in your body increases lightness and softness and allows for the other elements to come together and to exist.

Air

The second element is air. Ask yourself, what are the qualities of air? Air moves and is the element of movement and kinetic energy. With the introduction of movement, air allows for the sensation of touch. Air possesses the qualities of weightlessness. It is mobile, cool, dry, porous, and subtle. Air produces the action of touch and vibration and is anything that is dry and airy. Air creates gas, gassiness or bloating in the body. Toast, cookies, and cabbage are prime examples of foods that naturally possess a high level of the air element. Air increases dryness, right? When you walk into a bathroom in most public places nowadays to wash your hands and look around for paper towels, what do you normally find lined up on the wall; electric hand dryers. The action and qualities of those machines are of similar actions and qualities of the air element. If you had dry skin, would you want to place your skin under one of those high-powered hand dryers? If your skin is dry, why would you want to consume foods that possess similar qualities? Fall is the time of year in most areas of the country possessing similar qualities, thus automatically increasing the likeness within our minds and bodies.

Fire

The sensation and movement of air creates friction. Friction allows for the manifestation of the next universal element, fire. Fire is hot, produces heat and is always moving upward. We have all heard the saying that "heat rises...!" The qualities of fire are hot, sharp, subtle, weightless, and rough. It possesses the action of radiation of heat and light and facilitates form, color and temperature. Fire is anything combustible, as well as spicy and hot. Some examples of foods we eat that possess an abundance of the fire element are chilies, cloves, cinnamon, and pepper. In the body, the fire element is responsible for digestion and metabolism, as well as the glow and color of the skin. Fire is responsible for not only the transformation of foods but also the transformation of thoughts and sensory input. Someone who possesses a high level of the fire element within their mind is often referred to as being "sharp" or "bright." This element allows for the quick transformation of information, thus facilitating the ability to think quickly and most times accurately.

Water

The heat from fire produces the manifestation of condensation, which thus forms water. Water always moves in a downward direction with gravity. The qualities of water are oily, moist, cool, soft, and sticky. It possesses the attributes of cohesion and lubrication and facilitates fluidity and taste via saliva in the body. It is anything that is liquid or fluid or watery. Common examples, of course, are drinks, melons, cucumber and celery. Water increases smoothness, coolness and softness. Ask yourself, does the recommended consumption of eight, 8oz. glasses of water every day make sense for someone who naturally possesses higher amounts of the water element? Water, plus water, added with more water equals what...?

Earth

The fifth and final universal element is earth. Earth is solid, unmoving and stagnant. Earth is stable and very dense. Since the earth element is more visible and can be touched, it is the least subtle of all the five elements. Earth possesses the qualities of heaviness, roughness and is slow. It is resistant and facilitates fragrance, odor and shape. Earth is heavy and solid. Examples of common foods that we consume that has high levels of the earth element are fried foods, meats, cheeses and bananas. The earth element in the body is responsible for solidity and stability, and in excess can easily lead to obesity. When the earth element is maintained and cultivated, it can lead to an increase of muscle mass growth, compassion and understanding. I am willing to bet that most of the professional bodybuilders who compete for their sports top prize possess higher levels of the earth element within their natural dispositions, as well as consuming massive amounts of foods possessing higher levels of the earth element.

Understood and incorporated correctly, this knowledge becomes a powerful method for realizing the way we as humans interact with our environment, foods, and even our thoughts. The elegance of this science lies in the simplicity of its concepts and the effective tools it provides for one to be able to live a healthy, balanced life. We will talk more about the five elements and strengthen our understanding of them as we delve further into this work, but for now, rest assured that you are a few pages away from never having to worry about what's the latest diet fad and if that will work for you!

Understanding the Real You

Theory of Similarities and Differences –
"Common features and characteristics lead to growth. Differences or specialties in characteristics lead to division and degeneration or depletion."
- **Charaka sutra sthana, Chapter 26, verse 45**

सामान्यमेकत्वकरं, विशेषस्तु पृथक्त्वकृत्।

तुल्यार्थता हि सामान्यं, विशेषस्तु विपर्यय:॥४५॥

Samanyamekatvakaram, visheshstu prathakatvakrit, tulyartha hi samanayam, visheshastu viparyaye

In order for the five universal elements to exist, react, and create, they need to become unified. Working together as one to create and destroy, they form a unique collection within the human body and mind. This special collection of the five universal elements within each of us creates and constitutes our unique body-type or unique mental make-up, or in Ayurveda, *dosha*.

Knowing and understanding this special collection of the five elements is crucial in understanding what foods you'll need to eat, what exercises you'll need to engage in, which career best suits you, which climate to live, and how to return yourself to a state of health on the days you're not feeling well. Yes, this unique collection makes you what and who you are and is unwavering throughout your current life. The rare collection of the elements was set forth at the time of your conception, and many factors such as was your mother eating a hotdog or was your dad upset over the big game played an important role in creating you. This specialized collection is universal, unchanged, and will remain constant forever. This is the good news. The bad news is that the state of your body and mind can become vitiated at any time and for an endless number of reasons. It is this knowledge of understanding how, what, why and when becomes so important. Knowing and understanding this crucial information will not only tell you how to dress in the winter, but will tell you what to eat, when to eat, and even how to eat. Knowing your *dosha* is more important than knowing your name. After all... your name can be changed.

The unique combination of the five elements in the body is classified as *vata*, *pitta*, and *kapha*. In Sanskrit, the "a" is most always pronounced as a long "a," as is father. *Vata*, (pronounced "vah-tuh") is created from space and air. *Pitta*, (pronounced "pit-uh") is comprised of fire and water. *Kapha*, (pronounced "kuh-fuh") is created from water and earth. Now, you must understand that even though you might be predominantly one *dosha*, we all have certain levels of all three *doshas* inherent within our minds and bodies. These collections are so rare and so unique, and though you may be classified as the same as your son or your grandmother, you are not the same. You'll never be the same. Now, does this mean if you have a family of five, you will need to cook five separate meals? It would be a good idea in theory and though cooking is very therapeutic and fun for most, it does not. A dash of a simple spice or the addition of one extra ingredient can change the landscape of the meal making it a balancing or unbalancing meal for you. We will go into specifics later on in this work, but for now, let us take a closer look at the three body-types so you can understand what they are, how they operate and how they play a crucial role in your creation and well-being.

Any imbalances of these elemental combinations is the direct cause of physical disease - they are the prime disease-causing factors (contaminants). Secondary factors in the disease process, like body tissues, toxins and waste materials are the products of, or dependent upon, an imbalance in the *doshas*. It is difficult to translate the precise meaning of *dosha*. It is often translated as "biological type" or physical constitution. This definition allows for a simple and easy understanding of the concept. The original definition of *dosha*, however, is more complex. In Sanskrit, *dosha* can be defined as the literal meaning of "that which contaminates, or fault." In essence, the state of the *doshas* may be considered the pathogenic factors, or disease-causing agents in the body and mind. An imbalance of *vata, pitta,* and *kapha* causes disease in the body and in the mind.

One way we need to think of and define the three doshas is as the three biological energies of *vata, pitta,* and *kapha*. I know this view may be hard to swallow for a lot of you hardcore Westerners, I know it was for me. In time, you will begin to not only marvel over the simplicity of this philosophy, but it will soon begin to change the paradigm of your thinking. Once you do, the way you view yourself, your diet, career and your daily routine will never again be the same. Like any learned skill or behavior it will take time for you to think from this state of mind. Doing so will allow you to witness just how easy it can be to live in a state of health and joy.

Vata

Space and air, never again will your view of these two things be so narrow-minded. They are the first elements of creation and due to their unique properties and characteristics, they are two of the most important elements. As we speak of the characteristics of *vata,* recall the qualities of air and space. Knowing and understanding this will be the deciding factor when choosing what to have for lunch tomorrow, how to dress for your 8-year-old's soccer game on Sunday, or even if you should accept that promotion and move to "the windy city."

Anyone with a predominance of *vata* the body-type displays physical and emotional characteristics linked to the elemental qualities of space and air. Typically, they're very active, mobile, restless and energetic. They have fast metabolisms, so are often thin with little muscle development and protruding joints that may make cracking noises. Their skin is often found to be dry, rough and thin with visible veins. Why, because air moving in space has a drying effect. Something that is dry will cause dryness. Dryness will cause cracking of the skin and dehydration. Are you starting to see the connection?

The movement of air is irregular; therefore, their sleeping, eating and daily routines are predominantly irregular and erratic, with appetite and sexual desire varying between extremes. Is it their fault? Well, if you remember the literal definition it is their "fault," but it is certainly not their error or mistake.

Are you someone who sleeps lightly for no apparent reason, or do you have a tendency towards insomnia? Or perhaps you are someone who is talkative and really enjoys all forms of communication. As the seasons change and the air becomes cooler and the days grow shorter, do you welcome or fear this type of change? How you answer this question will help give you an idea of which body-type you might actually be.

Mentally and emotionally a *vata* person is rapid. They gather information and display emotions quickly. By determining swifty whether they like or dislike something, they always seem to be changing their minds. While they are rapid learners and are usually intellectual, their retention is poor. Money is spent quickly and impulsively. Demonstrating high creativity and innovation, they have tendencies to being sensitive or to experience hypersensitivity.

Individuals with this nature are introspective, shy, modest and often lack confidence. They are often unsettled and impatient, but very flexible and adaptable to change. People who are primarily *vata dosha* often feel anxious, worried, or stressed - especially in unfamiliar, cramped or noisy environments. They are most likely to be loners or non-conformists.

Now, if you or someone you know displays any of these characteristics, it does not necessarily mean that your nature is that of *vata dosha*. It can mean many things. You could be another body-type, but for whatever reason there has been an increase of the air and space element, causing a vitiation or excess of the *vata dosha*. Remove the excess stimuli and the balancing of your *dosha* should return to its normal state, which is called *prakruti* in Ayurveda.

Don't worry, we will not only uncover your unique body type, but you will have the power to change the above equation to offset any imbalance you may be experiencing, regardless of its causative factors. Knowing this and how to apply it will become your life's most important tool, for it can help you build a strong foundation of health and greater well-being.

Pitta

The *pitta* dosha is created from fire and water, though primarily fire. Someone who is predominantly *pitta* displays inherently the elemental characteristics of this *dosha*. They typically house a medium build, but with greater muscular development than that displayed by the *vata* type. They exhibit skin that is soft and warm, and they have a lot of body heat and often perspire excessively. Their hair is thin and often reddish or blond, and they may experience premature graying, baldness or excessive hair loss. Their skin flushes easily and they often have many freckles and moles. They are more prone to acne, and they burn easily in the sun, especially during the first few exposures to increased sunlight.

Since fire is hot and robust, a *pitta* person usually displays strong hunger and sexual appetite. Do you know or are you someone who feels the need to constantly eat, but under normal circumstances hardly ever gains a pound? This is a prime indicator of the *pitta dosha*. Increased sexual experiences or tendencies can often create an elevation of the fire element, thus creating a vitiation of the *pitta dosha*. So, cool it with the sex!

Their sleep is moderate and not easily disturbed. They have a strong pulse and its beat and frequency is stable. Individuals with *pitta dosha* usually speak loudly and passionately and often dominate the conversation. They have an aversion to hot weather, sunlight and heat and their eyes are sensitive to light. They normally have impaired or excellent eyesight. Thankfully, I was blessed with the latter, well, until I turned 43.

In behavior and temperament they are extroverted and love to be the focus of attention. Although, they can control their emotions, they may become irritable, angry and judgmental under stressful situations. Money is prudently managed. They're decisive, aggressive, ambitious and determined, often aspiring to positions of leadership. Enjoying competitive sports and games, either as spectators or participant, is often their passion. Their intelligence is high and they have good insight and a keen sense of discrimination. Being self-confident with an overly active entrepreneurial spirit, makes them successful in various forms of business ownership.

Fire is unmistakable and witnessing the same qualities in either one's behavior and or physiology is no different. Become one with who you are, understand it and cultivate it. Do not destroy or mask or dull the natural tendencies that makes you that which you are. If you are quick, witty and very creative, look for career fields or pastimes that will allow you to utilize these unique abilities.

If you do and do so earnestly, you'll be considered nothing less than an expert in your field. It is who you are... and that is a marvelous thing.

Kapha

People with a predominance of the *kapha dosha* tend to possess a heavy and solid, or large build. They have a tendency towards being overweight. They can gain weight easily, though they possess high muscle development (plump and round). After all, if you take a moment to consider the qualities of the earth and water elements, then it is not hard to see why they possess natural strength and endurance, as well as have a tendency towards weight gain and obesity when out of balance.

The skin of a *kapha* individual is thick, smooth and moist with few wrinkles. Their complexion is clear, fair or pale, and their hair is oily, thick and wavy. They have large and strong teeth, which are white and well-formed. There is no mistaking the true beauty of someone who is *kapha* by their full, thick hair and their radiant, soft skin. If Maybelline could bottle the essence of *kapha*, it would be an instant worldwide bestseller!

Kapha type individuals have a moderate or low appetite and a slow, and sometimes sluggish digestion. They enjoy eating gourmet or luxury foods (that appeal to taste and smell) or buying and preparing food. In movement and activity, they tend to be slow and methodical with excellent endurance. They can be sluggish and lethargic, though, and have a hard time getting motivated. They are prone to sleeping heavily and excessively. Their pulse is slow, steady and regular. They have a pleasant appearance and voice.

In behavior and temperament, they prefer familiar surroundings, traditions, and they love their steadfast routines. The *kapha* types are slow to learn but have excellent memories. Money is hoarded (or they are thrifty) and they are good, stable providers. Typically, they are serene and tranquil, and their emotions are slow to become excited or aroused. By being sentimental, nostalgic and romantic in nature, they normally prefer to be in a committed relationship. In addition, they are highly tolerant and forgiving. By possessing medium intelligence, they prefer to be guided or directed. They prefer to belong to a group, club or community and cling to their family or familial associations. These, of course, like the tendencies of all three *doshas*, are examples of the traits more commonly found to be exhibited by each *doshic* type. Having a proper assessment from a trained Ayurvedic practitioner is the only true way to discover your *dosha* and its current state (*vikriti*).

Your given elemental nature or dosha is what it is, and no court or judge can change it for you. For instance, if you wish to acquire *pitta* qualities in order to run this country, you cannot do so by eating foods high in the fire and water elements. By doing so, you will only disturb your primary *dosha*, and will inevitably see the imbalance manifest itself as some illness or disease (most likely a common *pitta* imbalance). Changing your nature through acquiring positive qualities and minimizing negative temperamental characteristics, is the role of the mind.

When healthy, you are instinctively attracted to foods and activities similar in elemental composition to your *prakriti* (God-given constitution). When you are sick and the elements are unbalanced, you are attracted to those foods opposite in nature. For example, if you are suffering from a cold or chest congestion (due to an imbalance in the *kapha dosha*), you will be attracted to foods of a like nature, such as meats and dairy products. You should choose, however, to avoid those foods that possess the same qualities as the manifestation of the imbalance itself. Examples of foods with inherently high levels of the earth and water elements are dairy products, heavy and oily foods and meats. Ask yourself, do you think it is a good idea to eat heavy, oily cold foods while you're suffering from a sinus infection which exhibits high levels of mucus? But why not avocados? Avocados are healthy, aren't they? After all, they're considered a superfood, right? The qualities of the avocado are cold, oily and gooey. Those qualities will heighten and increase symptoms such as phlegm, mucus and congestion in the lungs. What should you consume when you have a cold? Keep reading, and you will not only find out what, but will soon understand why.

Seasons, a Time of Change

While growing up in New England, the change of the seasons meant only two things: I had to change what I wore, and I either had to shovel the driveway or mow the lawn. The changing of the seasons now brings forth an entirely new meaning for me... and it should for you as well. Ever experience the same illnesses around the same time of year? Ever wonder why? From this point forward, seasonality is something which you'll need to start placing a higher importance on if you want to stay balanced and healthy throughout the year. Each *dosha* or body type has a corresponding season. The constitution or make-up of spring is like *kapha*, summer is similar in nature to *pitta*, vata is that of fall and winter is the season of *vata* and *kapha*.

With the changing of the seasons you need to start thinking about the following:

- Change of wardrobe
- Change of diet
- Change of activity
- Detoxification

We have a tendency to ignore all of the above except to change what we are wearing. We go from wearing boots to sneakers and sandals and back again, but most ignore what food they eat and in which activities to participate. You should opt to choose foods of a balancing nature or that of an opposite quality. As an example, someone who is *pitta* shouldn't consume the jalapeño stuffed peppers at the family cookout mid-summer. Rather, they should choose the mint and mango salad instead. As a generalized guide, I will go into each season in greater detail, but remember your specific and unique plan is something we can create together at the end of this work. For now, however, I will give a general description of each season and how they relate to the *tridoshas*.

Spring

The tastes you'll need to consume the most during springtime are foods with the bitter and astringent taste. Foods slightly pungent in most areas are acceptable. The goal of the spring diet is to burn off or eliminate the excess qualities of earth and water that have accumulated during the colder months of the winter. Ginger, turmeric, and cinnamon can be excellent additions to any meal, while opting for porridge or oatmeal-like dishes for breakfast. During this time you will want to avoid foods similar in qualities as to those which you are trying to get rid of; water and earth. You will want to avoid consuming cold and heavier foods, and though yogurt offers a digestional benefit due to its probiotic nature, limit the consumption of dairy during this time of year. You will also want to avoid taking naps after meals as this activity increases the earth and water qualities and can lead to undigested foodstuff (*ama*) unknowingly forming in your body. Ayurveda considers *ama* to be the root cause of all disease. *Ama* is the accumulation of food byproducts which your body was unable to effectively digest, assimilate and eliminate. By paying attention to easy to control factors like taking naps after meals during the springtime months, you'll be able to greatly reduce the amount of undigested waste in your body. I will go into *ama* and how to avoid it in greater detail in a coming chapter, but for now let's move on with looking at the importance of seasonality.

Summer

Summer is hot and can be extremely humid in most areas. So during the fiery months of the summer, it is common sense then to avoid spicy foods and choose foods which are inherently cooler in nature. The sweet taste is cooling, so during the summer, you will need to consume foods that are naturally sweet (always avoid sugary and highly refined foods). This is the time of the year to bathe in yogurt, so to speak. Mango Lassi; a yogurt-based drink prepared with mango and cardamom, is an excellent choice at the end of most meals. This sweet treat is balancing, very tasty and an excellent digestive aid. Consuming foods higher in the water element also becomes important; hence why watermelons and other melons are excellent summer choices and are harvested at this time of year. Coconut water is both cooling and very hydrating. Mint, cilantro and all forms of coconut are cooling and excellent choices. It will be a goal of your meal creation to base your recipes using predominantly cooling foods. Stay hydrated, stay out of the hot sun, and opt for cooling water-based activities, especially if you are the *pitta* type or suffering from a like imbalance.

Fall

As the crisp and drier winds of the fall blow about, the *vata* type will need to be most concerned. Fall is the *vata* time of year. Since *vata* is composed of space and air, this becomes the time of the year where the *vata* type will need to be the most disciplined. This is so important that even the time of day to consume meals is different for each season and each *dosha*. Do not worry, this is something that we will specifically cover in your reader-specific version of this work. Lunchtime should be earlier in the day, at about noon time, and NO salads! During the fall, you'll want to consume a *vata* pacifying diet. Regular consumption of the sweet, sour and salty foods are wise choices. Now, of course, this does not mean you cannot have the occasional lettuce (bitter & astringent) wrap, but let's try to make a conscious effort this coming fall to reduce these foods. Avocados... I'll say it again, avocados! They are not only an excellent choice during the fall, but they are highly nutritious as well. They are heavy, oily and are high in fiber. Due to these qualities, avocados get things moving! Ghee is one of the best things you can consume, not only during the fall or autumn but any time of the year. Ghee, or clarified butter, is very nourishing and easy to digest. Ghee promotes vitality. Soups are easy to digest, so they become great choices on that windy Halloween night. Choose a warmer and spicier soup if it is colder. Warmer baths and self-massage (*abhyanga*) with calming oils can also provide a balancing effect, not to mention they feel amazing.

Winter

Brrr...! Winter is cold in most areas, and the body uses more energy to produce heat and to keep heat locked inside of the body. The spring and summer are times of release. Keeping your digestive fire burning hot is important all year long, but this will be one of your main goals during the winter months. During the colder times of the year you will want to consume warmer and more nourishing foods. If you have a slower digestion (*kapha*, in general) you will want to consume foods which enhance your digestive capacity, like ginger and avoid difficult to digest foods such as meats and cheeses. Winter is the time of year which inherently possesses higher levels of the earth and water elements, so the *kapha* type will need to become more disciplined around Christmas. Is it a coincidence that Santa is a bit heavy?

Warm and spicy soups and nourishing kitchari meals are best. Foods or spices which get things moving are highly recommended, like cayenne pepper (*pitta's* proceed cautiously here). Dinner should be consumed earlier in the day as we have a natural tendency to sleep earlier due to the fact that it gets darker much sooner in the day. Remember, seasons change, this is inevitable. A good tip; each time you change your type of footwear, change your diet as well!

The Taste of it

"The strength, complexion, immunity etc. of a living system is under the control of diet, which in turn is under the control of six rasas"
— Susruta Samhita, Sutra Sthana, Chapter 1, verse 28

एक जीवित प्रणाली की ताकत, जटिलता, प्रतिरक्षा आदि आहार के नियंत्रण में है, जो बदले में छह रसों के नियंत्रण में है

"Sarvam dravyam Panchabhautikam"
i.e. all creation arises out of five great elements known as mahabhutas.

If I were to ask, could you name the six tastes? I have asked this question countless times in numerous classes, seminars and lectures. Surprisingly, over 90% of the people get the same exact 4 out of the 6 every time; sweet (of course), salty, sour and bitter... but what are the last two? According to Ayurveda, they are pungent and astringent. You're probably asking yourself why is he talking about what food tastes like. What does this have to do with being healthy, other than the fact that most know too many sweets and too much salt is unhealthy for you... or is it?

All foods, everything you eat and drink is classified in several different ways. As an example, they are classified by their nutritional value, their effect on the mind and body, whether they are heating or cooling, as well as by their taste. Ayurveda recognizes the six tastes as playing a vital role in the health of our physiology and overall well-being. The six tastes, as mentioned above are as follows:

1. Sweet
2. Sour
3. Salty
4. Bitter
5. Pungent
6. Astringent

Let us take a moment and look more closely at the six tastes and how they relate to your overall health. Everyone, as well as that chair over there and your car, all possess a unique and very specific combination of the five universal elements (*panchamahabhutas*). Each of the six tastes are no different, and each taste is comprised of a precise combination of space, air, fire, water and earth. We will also look at which organs in the body relates most to each taste, as well as what area of the tongue has a greater capacity for sensing each of the six tastes. With that said, however, the entire tongue can sense eat individual taste but not as effectively as the separate seats of the tongue.

Sweet

The sweet taste is comprised of the water and earth elements. Now, when I refer to sweet, I am not only talking about the sugary and highly processed taste most of us are accustomed to consuming, but rather foods containing natural sugars. As an example, beets and carrots, though are classified as a vegetable and most would not consider them to be a yummy treat, are both naturally sweet. All meat, including fish, pork, chicken and red meat are inherently sweet. Wheat is also sweet. So it is easy to see that the sweet taste will increase the levels of *kapha*. Protein, unknowingly, is not the only reason bodybuilders crave and consume mass amounts of animal products; the earth element can lend to a muscular physique. An excessive amount, as well as a deficiency in the sweet taste influences the body and mind accordingly. Here is a brief list of benefits to consuming the proper amount of the sweet taste:

- Strengthening
- Nutritive tonic
- Relieves thirst
- Cools and relieves burning sensations
- Beneficial to hair & skin
- Nourishing to most bodily tissues
- An aphrodisiac
- Promotes pregnancy & lactation
- Beneficial to mucous membranes: lining the mouth, the lungs, the GI tract, the urinary tract, and the reproductive system

The sweet taste is highly overindulged, as you can most likely imagine, mainly due to its abundance in today's more commonly processed foods (via highly processed sugars). The salty taste is the second most commonly consumed taste in the Standard American Diet (S.A.D). The addictive aspects of sugar is an issue that not only do we need to strictly monitor, but it is something that we as a nation need to address. In excess, the sweet taste can lead to numerous imbalances and manifestation, not only within the body, but within the mind as well. Here is a brief list of the more common manifestations:

- Distinguishes the digestive fire, thus diminishing appetite
- Increases mucus
- Promotes congestion, thus leading to coughs & coldness in the body
- Increases swelling of the lymph glands
- Flaccidity
- Laziness
- Excess weight gain
- Edema
- Increases of greed behaviors (mind)
- Dampness

Organ of Affinity - upper area of the lungs and the thyroid gland

Area of Tongue Detection - front center, tip of the tongue

The sweet taste, though appealing to the taste buds, has become an epidemic of vast proportions in today's fast-paced world of 1,000 calorie lattes and fast food meals. We will look at how to properly manage your consumption of sugar as well as the sweet taste in Part Two of this book.

Salty

The salty taste is comprised of the fire and water elements. Which *dosha* is consistent with fire and water...that's right, *pitta*. Examples of the salty taste are of course table salt, as well as seaweed. Salt increases heat and can increase or aggravate *pitta* and *kapha* doshas (in higher amounts). Sprinkling salt on a salty tortilla chip after you've eaten a few extra spicy wings will NOT pacify the heat. It will only increase its effect. If you undertake this challenge and your mouth is on fire, opt for a glass of milk or a spoonful of cottage cheese instead. Below is a list of a few of the more commonly manifested positive effects of the salty taste upon your physiology:

- Balances the *vata dosha*
- Imparts softness within the body
- Causes a downward movement of the doshas
- Distributes throughout the body quickly
- Helps excretion of an excess of the *kapha dosha*
- Can overpower and dominate all other tastes

An excess of the salt element in the body can manifest as the following symptoms (though not limited to this list):

- Increases the *pitta* & *kapha* doshas
- Vitiation of the blood
- Causes excess thirst
- Degeneration of muscle tissue
- Skin inflammatory issues
- Infertility, impotence (in excess)
- Excessive graying and hair loss
- Gastritis
- Aggravates eczema (commonly a *pitta* imbalance)

Organ of Affinity - kidneys

Area of Tongue Detection - rear, outer edges of the tongue

Qualities (*guna*) - heavy, hot, oily, and has a downward movement

Salt, as all of the six tastes, becomes important to correctly incorporate into your diet at the appropriate times of year. Monitoring your salt intake becomes important due to the fact that most processed foods possess high levels of salt (sodium). All forms of salt are considered to possess the elemental factors of the salty taste, including sea salt and pink himalayan.

Sour

The sour taste is comprised of the fire and earth elements. Now since there is no one single dosha which is comprised of exactly fire and earth, the sour taste will/can aggravate the *pitta* and *kapha doshas*, but at the same time will pacify the *vata dosha*. Examples of sour foods are anything fermented and most acidic foods and wine. Yogurt is sour as are pickles and lemons. Pickles, because they're both sour and salty are aggravating to a *pitta* person, but because of its warming nature can burn off the coldness and dampness of any excess earth and water. Here is a brief list of the benefits of incorporating the sour taste into your diet:

- Balances the vata *dosha*
- Heightens digestion by increasing mouth salivation
- Cleanses the oral cavity
- Induces sweating

- Promotes overall heart health
- Helps eliminate excessive urine in the bladder
- Improves the movement of fluids within the body's channels
- Satitates the mind
- Acts as a laxative
- Retains fluids in tissues

Consuming an excess of the sour taste, just as in consuming anything in excess, can lead to disturbances within the *doshas*. Here are a few manifestations of an increase of the sour taste:

- Increases *pitta* & *kapha doshas*
- Increases inflammatory conditions
- Causes excessive thirst
- Destabilizes the body
- Causes burning sensations in the throat and chest
- Dries out the mucus membranes
- Hyperacidity
- Heartburn
- Ulcerative colitis
- Diarrhea

Organ of Affinity - lungs

Area of Tongue Detection - front outer edges of the tongue

Qualities (*guna*) - heavy, oily, cold and often difficult to digest

The sour taste is more commonly consumed from dairy products, however, there are other sources of the sour taste such as tomatoes, which we may want to incorporate into your diet. We will, of course, take a look at your specific situation in your customized version of this work.

Bitter

The bitter taste is comprised of the air and space elements. An example of the bitter taste is black coffee; yes, please! The elements of air and space is what comprises the *vata dosha,* so an excessive consumption of the bitter taste will aggravate *vata dosha.* Are you starting to see the connection here and how everything within and around us is all inter-related?

The bitter taste, though not the most sought-after of the tastes, is one that is very distinguishable. It aggravates *vata* in excess, but balances *pitta* and *kapha doshas.* When consumed in proper amounts according to your constitution, it can lead to numerous health benefits. The following is a brief list:

- Balances *pitta* & *kapha dosha*
- Excellent detox benefits; scrapes fat and toxins
- Appetite stimulant
- Kills germs
- Removes parasites from GI tract
- Relieves heat

- Helps eliminate ama (undigested food matter)
- Purifies blood
- Cleanses the liver
- Relieves burning, itching and swelling; especially from the skin
- Relieves intestinal gas
- Promotes peristalsis,
- Digestive tonic

Even despite its many health benefits, it can lead to imbalances within the *doshas* if consumed in excess or during inappropriate times of the year. Here are some of the common symptoms and manifestation caused from an excess consumption of the bitter taste:

- Aggravates the *vata dosha*
- Causes nausea
- Weakens the kidneys & lungs
- Emaciation and dryness of tissues
- Dryness of mouth
- Weight Loss
- Fainting & unconsciousness (in excess)

Organ(s) of Affinity - pancreas, liver and spleen

Area of Tongue Detection - center area of the tongue

Qualities (*guna*) - cold, dry, light and it also has a descending or downward movement

The bitter taste is one that should be diminished for all *doshic* types during pregnancy. Now, ladies, this is not a prescription to stop consuming healthy greens, it simply becomes something that you'll want to monitor during pregnancy more so due to the potential for increased exposure to toxins. Washing and properly preparing and cooking your fresh produce becomes an even more important act when pregnant and nursing.

Pungent

The pungent taste, or as more commonly known as spicy or hot, is comprised of air and fire. What does fire need to burn hot and bright...? Any foods that are spicy, hot and warming are pungent. Some examples are cinnamon, cayenne pepper, and clove. The pungent taste aggravates the *pitta* body-type the most. Since I am the *pitta* type, this is the taste I am most attracted to, you might know this to be true as well. The pungent taste aggravates the *pitta dosha* (can also aggravate the *vata dosha*) and is balancing for the *kapha dosha*.

Pungencency is created via the presence of aromatic and volatile oils, resins and mustard glycosides, which stimulates the tissues and nerve endings of the mouth, thus providing the sensation of heat or spiciness. The pungent taste due to its warming qualities obviously provides heat and increases circulation in the body, however, it also cleanses the mouth and clarifies the organs of sense. Here are a few more positive manifestations which can occur via the proper consumption of the pungent taste:

- Balances the *vata dosha*
- Stimulates tongue
- Improves digestion, absorption and elimination
- Helps eliminate intestinal worms
- Induces lacrimation and secretions from nose and mouth
- Cleanses oral cavity
- Sharpens sense organs
- Eliminates moisture, congestion and stagnation in the body
- Absorbs liquid
- Stimulates heart
- Keeps the mind sharp and bright
- Aids in weight loss
- Has scraping effect over the body channels

Below is a brief list of negative manifestations that can occur due to an overconsumption of the pungent taste:

- Increases burning sensations
- Causes fainting
- Induces bleeding
- Increases inflammation
- Causes excessive thirst
- In excess can cause fatigue
- Causes heartburn & peptic ulcers

- Diarrhea & constipation
- Colitis
- In excess can cause mental confusion and malaise
- Aggravates *pitta*, in excess can aggravate *vata* due to increased dryness
- Diminishes sperm count
- Sexual debility in both men and women, whereas in females it can kill the ova

Organ(s) of Affinity - stomach and heart

Area of Tongue Detection - center, behind the sweet receptors and in front of the bitter receptors

Qualities (*guna*) - hot, dry, sharp, penetrating and moves in an upward direction

The pungent taste can easily increase levels of the fire element, especially during the hot and dry months. During the summertime, a person who is primarily *pitta* or suffering from an increase of the *pitta dosha* will want to avoid the pungent foods in areas of the US such as Arizona, western part of Texas and southern part of New Mexico. Ginger (cooked), despite being warming and possessing higher amounts of the fire element, does not aggravate the *pitta dosha* in small amounts. This, of course, is a person-specific case when managing the amounts of ginger and like foods.

Astringent

The astringent taste is the least known out of all of the six tastes. It is one of the more lacked tastes in our diet here in the US, and is one of the tastes that may take greater conscious effort to successfully incorporate into your diet. The astringent taste is comprised of earth and air. Anything containing tannins, like black tea is astringent. Aloe vera and aloe vera juice are also astringent, though they do possess the bitter quality as well. Most leafy greens are both bitter and astringent. Regular consumption can help pacify or fill the need for this ever so important taste and quality. Let's examine a few of the more common positive manifestation which stem from the astringent taste:

- Pacifying to the *pitta* & *kapha doshas*
- Promotes clotting, this inhibits bleeding
- Decongestant
- Cleanses the mucus membranes
- Absorbs excess moisture
- Scraps excess fat
- Improves absorption
- Binding effect for loose stool
- Healing to wounds

When consumed in excess, especially for the *vata dosha*, certain physical and also mental manifestations can occur as shown below:

- Aggravating for *vata dosha*
- Increases dryness

- Can cause choking sensations in excess
- Gas, bloating and distention in the G.I. tract
- Emaciation and convulsions in excess
- Excessive thirst
- Stiffness
- Coagulation & excessive clotting of the blood
- Stagnation
- Insomnia
- Depression

Organ(s) of Affinity - colon

Area of Tongue Detection - back center of the tongue

Qualities (*guna*) - dry, cold, heavy and has a movement of drawing inward

If you are experiencing blockage of any kind, an increase of the astringent element can exacerbate the situation and/or condition. Manifestation and conditions due to an increase of astringency are more commonly found in someone who is vegetarian or who is flirting with veganism. Let's be honest, most people who are meat lovers, other than perhaps the potato, are not commonly falling victim to an excess of the astringent taste from over consumption of greens and other foods high in astringency. This is where knowing your specific *dosha* and its current state, added to your current lifestyle becomes crucial when trying to bring the body back into a balanced state and also in managing any situation of dis-ease.

Not only does each taste contain specific levels of each of the universal elements, they are also classified by their effect on the mind and body. For example, nutmeg which is dry, hot, and heavy, and its taste is astringent, will aggravate *pitta* and *kapha dosha*, but will pacify *vata*. So, knowing the effect that each taste has on your body is vitally important to keeping you balanced and healthy all year long. Honey, which is one of the few sweeteners that is warming, is a sweetener a person who is primarily *kapha dosha* can consume on a regular basis. The pungent taste is the hottest, followed by salty, bitter and sour. The coldest taste is bitter, followed then by astringent and sweet.

The six tastes are also classified by whether they are heavy or light. The *kapha dosha*, which is comprised of water and earth is the heaviest. Consuming heavier foods will increase these levels and could possibly create an imbalance. The heaviest taste is sweet, followed in order by salty and astringent. The lightest taste is bitter, followed by pungent and sour.

Lastly, the tastes can also be classified by whether they are moist or dry. The wettest taste is sweet, followed then by salty and sour. The driest taste is pungent, followed by bitter and astringent. I know it can seem like a daunting task to research, learn and remember the taste and quality of every food you eat and what body-type it will pacify or aggravate. Do not fear, that is what this work is all about. It is about YOU, and in the reader-specific option of this book we will not only examine the foods you are eating, but you will learn their properties, tastes and effects they're producing on your mind and body. Remember, I said at the start of the book that this work will be penned for you, by you and together we will create the ultimate lifestyle specifically for you!

Let's continue to delve further into the six tastes and their relationship to the human body, as well as the produced effect they have on the *doshas*.

Vata, which is created from space and air, is aggravated by the bitter and astringent taste, then by pungent. *Vata* is pacified by sweet and sour.

Pitta, which is comprised of fire and water, is most aggravated by the pungent and sour tastes, then followed by salty. The fire within us *pittas* is cooled by the bitter, astringent, and sweet tastes. Now, this is not a prescription for us to go out and eat a box of Twinkies, even despite the fact that many of you might be thrilled they've been brought back to the market (Yuck!).

Kapha, as you probably know by now, is formed from the water and earth elements. The *kapha* type is aggravated by the sweet, sour and salty tastes, and pacified by bitter and astringent tastes.

As you now see and hopefully understand, the taste of food is not limited to the perception or the distinguishing factor of its flavor. The taste of each ingredient you're consuming has a profound effect on your state of health. Managing their interplay of cause and effect upon your mind and body signifies one of the most important aspects in managing your health and the state of your mind and body. The pathogenic factors of the six tastes, even despite the fact that it is grossly overlooked here in this country, does not in any way negate its importance. Your custom diet as well as the remainder of this book will be built upon such principles.

Digestion, Do You Get it?

"Strength, health, longevity and vital breath are dependent upon the power of digestion including metabolism. When supplied with fuel in the form of food and drinks, this power of digestion is sustained; it dwindles when deprived of it."

- Charaka sutra sthana, Chapter 28, verse 342

बलमारोग्यमायुश्च प्राणाश्चाग्नौ प्रतिष्ठिताः| अन्नपानेन्धनैश्चाग्निर्ज्वलति व्येति चान्यथा ||३४२||

Balamarogyamayushcha pranashchangnau

pratishthita,annapanendhanaishchagnirjwalati vyeti chanyatha

We've all heard the saying, "you are what you eat." As you will soon come to understand, this adage is only telling us half of the truth. You've just learned that according to the Ayurvedic model, nutrition is based more so upon the 5 universal elements (*panchamahabhutas*), as we here in the West live by a caloric-based model of nutrition. Another very important distinction is the focus or the way we look at the foods we consume. You see, according to the conventional approach to health, we are mainly concerned about the calories and the nutritional aspects of our foods. In Ayurveda, even though they do place a slight importance upon our foods' nutritional components, they are more concerned with its qualities and digestibility. Here is a great example:

It was a cold day in the month of December, and I was standing behind the counter of one of my juice bars placing the produce order for the day when a young 29-year-old female walked into the store. She had a sullen look on her face, which some would mistake as being standoffish or bitchy and ordered our most commonly ordered raw juice; the "lean green." I struck up some small talk, and though she was very non-committal, she answered my questions with a half-assed smile. She wasn't nearly 4-5 sips into her green juice when she began opening up and slowly started saying more than a few words. The longer she stood there, the more she spoke. She began to speak of all the foods that she was allergic to and how she often experienced constipation. I know, TMI, right! She then went on to mention the frequency and severity of her headaches, as well as explain how her overall health affected her moods and how she always experienced a general feeling of lethargy. I was somewhat shocked, to say the least. She appeared young, was attractive, thin and athletic. Most would look at her and would think she was in perfect health; that couldn't be further from the truth. She mentioned that she had been to every doctor, specialist and even every holistic doctor in the state. After having spent over a full years' worth of her time and upwards of ten-thousand dollars, she wasn't any closer to a cure nor was she feeling any better. She sat there with discouragement on her face as she slurped down the last few sips of pulp.

This young lady's case was certainly not the only instance where someone would walk into my office or into one of my juice bars confessing that they were tired and felt sluggish, oftentimes to the point of not being able to sleep or even think clearly. People would sit there, sometimes for hours, expressing their disgust at not being able to lose any weight, having to take so many prescription medications, even despite having recently been eating healthier and exercising. Normally when I hear this, there are usually two main culprits at play; 1. their definition of what is "healthy" is not healthy for them. 2. their body and digestive system is impaired, and they're not properly digesting the food they eat. Not only are their digestive systems not properly digesting and assimilating the food they're consuming, but also, they are also not properly eliminating the waste. Well, if you're eating it, not processing it, and not all of it is being eliminated... then where is it going? To ensure good health and to maintain a balance of the three *doshas*, one must invite the "Shuns" over for each meal: digestion, assimilation, and elimination. If one of them cannot make it, so to speak, it is impossible to achieve a state of health. The longer the inconsistency of these three key factors exists, the more severe and more difficult the manifestation or manifestations will be to identify and correct. "Doc, I haven't pooped for five days... is that bad?" This is a question you never want to ask your doctor!

Everything in the universe is in a constant state of flux; ebb and flow. Our bodies are certainly not an exception to this rule. Our bodily organs and tissues are in a constant state of regeneration. They are continually being constructed and deconstructed. Even the cells of our bodies follow the principles of generation and regeneration. The important question you must ask yourself at this point, is how is this process happening?

In simpler terms, this process is twofold: the foods we consume and our body's ability to digest, assimilate and eliminate them. The energy, according to Ayurveda, that is responsible for the digestion is called, *agni*. *Agni* is such an important aspect in our health, that in certain Vedic cultures they worship the God of *Agni*. A key aspect to understand is that digestion happens on both the subtle and gross planes of manifestation. The digestive process has a few critical components that you must not only understand, but must also be able to effectively incorporate into your daily lifestyle. Here is a brief summary:

- *Agni* governs our strength, vitality, health, energy & luster
- *Agni* is the root of most imbalances, both in the mind & body
- Digests and processes foods
- Governs the process of waste
- *Agni* maintains your life force; when it is extinguished, the body withers & dies
- Balances the *doshas*; *vata* creates energy, *pitta* creates radiance & *kapha* forms strength

There is a three-stage process of digestion that must occur which takes approximately 4-6 hours to complete. The specifics of this, of course, is based upon the individual's *dosha*, the individual's age, and the strength of their digestive fire. Below is a list of the three stages of digestion[4]:

1. **Stage One** - occurs in the mouth and in the upper area of the stomach. Its duration normally takes 1.5 to 2.0 hours to complete. This stage of digestion is associated with the *kapha dosha*. During this aspect of digestion, saliva is secreted into the mouth which moistens the food, ultimately helping to make it more digestible. Saliva in the mouth begins to break down the food. The

---

[4] "The Digestive Process: An Ayurvedic Perspective | Banyan ...." 11 Jan. 2017, https://www.banyanbotanicals.com/info/blog-the-banyan-insight/details/the-digestive-process-an-ayurvedic-perspective/.

less the food is chewed, the greater the amount of saliva and time is needed to soften the food, so to speak. If you are tired after eating, it could represent that this process is taking too long or is not being effectively completed.

Stage Two - takes place in the lower area of the stomach and the small intestine. This aspect of digestion takes 2-3 hours, due to the fact that the body must literally, "re-cook" the food. Stage two relates to the *pitta dosha*, and it is during this process where pancreatic secretions begin to even further break down the food. Acid reflux and heartburn are imbalances that can often occur in this stage. A robust and brightly burning digestive fire increases the success of this stage.

Stage Three - occurs in the colon (large intestine). It is governed by the *vata dosha*, and takes approximately 1.5 hours to complete. In this stage the food particles are further broken down, and whatever unused parts are moved further along for elimination. Imbalances with this stage of digestion can manifest as gassiness, bloating and distention. It makes sense, since one of the governing elements of the *vata dosha* is air.

Bare with me for a few moments as I introduce you to some very uncommon sounding words and concepts. *Agni* is so critical in maintaining health that *agni* is classified in three categories, two of which have several sub-categories. The three categories are; *jatharagni, bhutagni and dhatu-agni*. *Jatharagni* governs the digestion of foods, *bhutagni* governs the digestion of the five elements, and *dhatu-agni* is responsible for the transformation of the energetic substances into the tissues[5]. *Dhatu*, in Sanskrit, means tissue[6]. The state of your *agni*, or digestive fire has 4 classifications; balanced (*sama agni*), variable (*vishama agni*), sharp (*teekshana agni*) and slow or weak (*mandu agni*). There is a relationship with the states of *agni* to each of the *tridoshas*, however, any one can experience any state of digestion for many different causative factors. During your assessment this is one area that together we will discover. Once the effectiveness and causative factors responsible for your digestive state are assessed, we will then proceed forth with this realization becoming the foundation for your diet and lifestyle regimen.

Each *agni* has its specific function in the transformation of the foods you consume into becoming what you witness in the mirror on a daily basis. The process of cooking, breaking down and assimilating the nutrients into a fluid-type substance is critical. This substance is then subsequently carried throughout the body where it nourishes and forms the tissues. The body is always nourished in a progressive order, the skin being the last organ nourished. This is not only important to understand for fully being able to understand the process of digestion, but it is also plays an important role when diagnosing the root cause of an imbalance. As an example, if you are experiencing anemia I know that the causative or pathogenic factors does not have to do with the reproductive organs simply because they are nourished and regenerated lower on the scale. This process is very similar to irrigation,

---

[5] "Physiological aspects of Agni - NCBI." https://www.ncbi.nlm.nih.gov/pmc/articles/PMC3221079/. Accessed 9 Jan. 2017.

[6] "Dhatu - Wikipedia." https://en.wikipedia.org/wiki/Dhatu. Accessed 19 Jan. 2017.

where each row of crops is provided with water in a successive flow. Here is the complete scale of nourishment according to Ayurveda in complete order:

1. Plasma / lymph
2. Red blood cell
3. Muscle
4. Fat
5. Bone
6. Bone marrow
7. Reproductive[7]

You are what you digested... 36 days ago

I mentioned at the start of this chapter that you are only what you consume and digest, but this process happens within a 36 day cycle. At the end of the 36 days, the entire process of digestion has created what Ayurveda refers to as *ojas*[8]. This energetic factor, or *Ojas*, contributes to the body's energy supply, thus helping to support healthy immune function. It is amazing how the body transforms the energy of our food into the energy of our bodies. All is energetic at the quantum level. I find it refreshing to witness how the concepts of Ayurveda are beautifully intertwined with the quantum philosophic model towards maintaining our well-being. I cover the quantum

---

[7] "The Seven Dhatus (tissues) in Ayurvedic Medicine."
https://www.ayurvedacollege.com/book/export/html/558. Accessed 6 Jan. 2017.

[8] "International Journal of Ayurveda and Pharmaceutical ... - OAJI." 10 Sep. 2017,
http://oaji.net/pdf.html?n=2019/1791-1549648335.pdf.

and spiritual model fully in another publication of mine, called "Law of One Mind".

The process of nourishing our body and its seven tissues above takes 36 days to complete. Now, even though the process takes 36 days, this is not a precise time table. Many factors can cause this to either be slightly slower or even slightly quicker than the 36 days. Factors such as your state of *agni* and time of year, just to name a few, can cause the formation of tissue to happen at varying rates. Here is the standard time table according to Ayurveda:

- **Day 1 - 5** - formation of plasma, serum and lymphatic fluid
- **Day 6 - 10** - formation of red blood cell
- **Day 11- 15** - formation of muscle tissue
- **Day 16 - 20** - formation of adipose tissue
- **Day 21- 25** - formation of bone
- **Day 26 - 30** - formation of bone marrow
- **Day 31 - 35** - formation of reproductive tissue
- **Day 36** - formation of *ojas*[9]

This process is subtle, meaning it is controlled by subtler aspects of your mind and its relationship to the Universal Intelligence that is the fabric upon which all is formed. Even though this intricate process is happening unbeknownst to your conscious awareness, it starts with a conscious choice as to what foods

---

[9] "The Digestive Process: An Ayurvedic Perspective | Banyan ...." 11 Jan. 2017, https://www.banyanbotanicals.com/info/blog-the-banyan-insight/details/the-digestive-process-an-ayurvedic-perspective/.

you consume. This may be one of the 2 remaining freedoms we as humans have left, of course, combined with our thoughts.

There are 5 keys to proper health

I have broken down all the aspects of the above into an easily understood and easy to incorporate 5 step process. We will go into your specific 5 step process in the customized version of this publication, but for now here are the guidelines is successive order:

1. The consumption of proper foods
2. The body's ability to digest or re-cook the foods
3. The body's ability to absorb the minute fragments of the food particles
4. The body's ability to assimilate nutrients from these specific food particles
5. The body's ability to eliminate waste from the food stuff

Ama, sticky yuckiness!

When the above process is not fully executed, *ama* is the end result. When your digestive state is currently residing in any of the four classifications, expect balanced (*sama agni*), *ama*... or a toxic byproduct is formed. *Ama* is undigested waste that the body has not utilized. *Ama* can be created by foods that the body absorbed but was not able to utilize, or foods that were simply undigested. If you could ever look at *ama*, it would look like a thick, gooey substance that can cause a slew of problems. If you are curious what it actually looks like, then before you brush your teeth in the morning or enjoy the morning's first cup of coffee, stick your tongue out and look in the mirror. What do you see? What color is it? That is *ama*! According to Ayurveda, *ama* is the root cause of all disease. It is that serious and maintaining proper digestion is just that important.

This undigested, sticky and gooey-stuff can cause, amongst many issues, created blockages of certain bodily channels. Obstructions in any of the bodily channels can lead to bodily disturbances, thus manifesting at some point as disease. It could develop as fibromyalgia or bronchitis. If not treated and left unattended it can manifest into life-threatening issues. The flow of energy throughout the bodily channels is also a very important aspect in maintaining a state of well-being. And although I am not going to get into specifics regarding these channels (*srotas*), they are nevertheless important. We will look more in depth at these energetic pathways in a later chapter.

The cause of *ama* or toxins in the body can be one or a combination of many. The first which we've just mentioned, is poor digestion. The yucky stuff can, however, form from overeating, eating heavy or processed foods, cold or iced foods, improper food combinations, contaminated foods, incompatible foods for one's dosha, poor eating habits (eating while driving or eating is a state of stress), sleeping before food is digested, eating before what you've eaten prior has not properly been digested, lack of proper exercise and believe it or not certain raw vegetables.

Typically, when each specific dosha is suffering from an imbalance, a direct correlation to one of the classifications of your digestive state is usually the cause. Here are the relationships[10]:

1. Variable digestion (*vishama agni*) results in *vata* imbalance
2. Sharp or over robust digestion (*teekshana agni*) results in *pitta* imbalance
3. Slow or sluggish digestion (*mandu agni*) results in *kapha* imbalance

Each classification of your digestive state, of course, will result in certain physical and mental manifestations. As an example, someone suffering from a slow or sluggish digestion (*mandu agni*) may experience any of the following:

1. Heaviness
2. Lethargy
3. Bloating & excess gas
4. Sour taste in mouth
5. White, thick coating on tongue
6. Fatigue
7. Blocked channels

If your digestion is overactive, sharp, or hyper (*teekshana agni*), you could experience any of the following:

1. Sour taste after belching
2. Vomiting greenish colored liquid
3. Hyper acidity

---

[10] "Physiological aspects of Agni - NCBI." https://www.ncbi.nlm.nih.gov/pmc/articles/PMC3221079/. Accessed 9 Jan. 2017.

4. Burning sensation in the throat or chest

If your digestion is variable and quick to change, you could experience any of the following:

1. Constipation
2. Excess gas
3. Bloating
4. Lower abdominal pain or distention
5. Prickling pain in the body

The root causes of *ama* can be plentiful and though I have covered most of the more common causative factors, I would like to introduce you to one that although does not fall under the scope of Ayurveda, it is certainly a potential cause of *ama* and various digestive disturbances.

There is a physiological outcome that is now known to conventional medicine called digestive leukocytosis. This unique physiological impairment was first brought to attention by a Suisse doctor by the name of Paul Kouchakoff. After cooking food above their critical temperature of approximately 188 degrees fahrenheit, Kouchakoff found that the body's response was an increase of white blood cells, suggesting that the process of cooking had bastardized the structure of the food as to where the human body interprets the food as being foreign and unrecognizable. His in depth study suggested, and by no means had he or am I suggesting a 100% raw food diet (raw food activists often misinterpret his findings to promote awareness of an all raw food diet), that if a certain percentage of your caloric intake is raw, the remaining calories could be consumed via cooked foods. Dr. Kouchakoff went on further to suggest by ensuring that if 10% of a meal's caloric intake was raw, that it severely reduced the body's white-blood-cell response, and the occurrence of leukocytosis was greatly reduced.[11] Though his findings may have a substantial scientific basis, by adding his theory with the importance of proper food combinations, we could develop a very critical aspect of digestion. I would love to see further studies done on this subject by combining Kouchakoff's theory with the philosophies of Ayurveda. I bet the results will not only supersede his original findings but create a food-based philosophy which can be the future premise of a healthy and balanced diet. A potential preventative for *ama* at the least, yes!

One of the main issues most of us have with digestion is a general ignorance towards it. I don't recall a single day in school where the importance of digestion was ever mentioned, let alone ways to evaluate a state of improper digestion and how to incorporate easy lifestyle changes to ensure it's working optimally. Now, with this said, I have noticed a major paradigm shift in the importance of eating healthier foods, especially with the ever-increasing popularity of the organic and non-GMO movements. This is such a positive trend, and I could not be any happier to see the banding of like-minded individuals like myself making such a positive change in the overall health of our country. Nevertheless, merely shoveling a handful of organic spinach in your mouth is not a cure-all for what is happening. Let's move forward and help spread the word on proper digestion by starting with properly

---

[11] "the influence of food cooking on the blood formula of man." https://pdfs.semanticscholar.org/0f9d/5c6e0dea63d68b05e86ca7e59a1622c7b5ab.pdf. Accessed 14 Jan. 2017.

identifying the root cause(s) of our own digestive issues, and then making simple everyday changes to effect long term results. Remember, change always starts with you!

I know this may seem not only daunting, but somewhat scary. Do not fear, however, because not only will we diagnose your current digestive state, but the art of eliminating *ama* and restoring proper digestion is not difficult at all. Actually, it is easy and systematic. I will cover the specific steps to eliminating *ama* and restoring your unique digestive state in the chapter titled "An Ancient Medicine for Modern Time", but for now, here are a few easy to incorporate activities you can start doing today: short and intermittent fasting, consume warm water with lemon first thing upon rising in the morning, incorporate herbs and spices with strong digestive benefits like fennel, cumin, black pepper and garlic.

We will look at the digestion process in depth later in this work, however, now that I've provided you with a deeper understanding of your overall digestion and its importance upon your health, I recommend that you start monitoring and engage in the art of self-observation. An unbiased look into your health is always the first line of defense - and always starts and ends with you.

Eat to Nourish, not to Diet!

"One should regularly take Shashtika (a kind of rice harvested in sixty days), Shali (rice), Mudga – green gram or Averrhoa carambola, rock salt, Amalaki (Amla – Emblica officinalis Gaertn), rain water, ghee, meat of animals dwelling in arid climates and honey"

— Charaka sutra sthana, Chapter 22, verse 12

षष्टिकाञ्छालिमुद्गांश्च सैन्धवामलके यवान्।

आन्तरीक्षं पयः सर्पिर्जाङ्गलं मधु चाभ्यसेत्॥१२॥

Shashtikayanchalimugdhashcha saidhavamlake yavaan,

antariksham payam sarpirjaangalam madhu chabhyaseta

My earliest recollection of the word "diet" brings me back to the year 1985. Back to the Future had just been released, and most of my days were spent playing hockey and collecting baseball cards. I recall rather vividly the day where I first understood the meaning of a diet, or so I thought. I was spending the night at a friend's house, and as we reluctantly made our way downstairs for dinner, I immediately took notice that everyone in his family was already seated at the dinner table except for his mother... her plate was still empty. I found this to be odd considering the fact that she was a 'big-boned" women. My confusion must have been clearly written all over my face because my buddy leaned over to whisper that his mom was on another diet, yet again. It was at that moment where skipping a meal, or better yet, caloric-reduction, became how I viewed dieting.

Today the word diet represents an entirely new meaning for me. Not only has its meaning changed considerably, but I also feel it is grossly misunderstood. It has become a tedious task that some of us must perform when we need to drop a few pounds, or even worse, an overused marketing term employed to lure the unsuspecting into falling victim for the latest weight-loss or health preventative trend. Don't take my word for it, test the theory. Ask ten people to define the word diet. Perhaps you may want to start by asking yourself. I feel that the word "diet" creates so much conjecture, that it either scares or excites. By definition, the word "diet" simply means the foods a species needs to survive and thrive. Most diets on the market today use the elimination technique, or rob Peter to pay Paul, so to speak. Cut the carbs and increase the fats. Cut the fat, and increase the carbs, or lower the sugar and increase the salt. The combinations are literally exhausting, leaving most people feeling confused and at the end unfulfilled, sicker and fatter.

I have researched and studied and have even run case studies on some of the most popular plans, magic pills and weight-loss fads from the past several years. The more I read and the further I've studied and tested, the more convinced I become that the philosophy upon which this book is written is the one true way to understand the term diet. If followed, not only does it work, but it also creates a system of long-term wellness and health. My intention here is not to impugn nor in any way demean the hard work or creativity of any of these systems or plans, but come on...the "Subway Diet?" I bet many diet-goers have shied away from this plan after it was released earlier this year that Subway had been using azodicarbonamide in their bread[12]. Azodicarbonamide is a dough conditioner used by bread processors to give the bread the perfect combination of airy and chewy, and it's a bleaching agent allowed in flour. Good, right? Not so much! It's also a blowing agent used by the rubber and plastics industries to make products like shoe soles and yoga mats springy. This so-called diet was most likely created by a high-level marketing executive within the Subway Corporation, and not by a certified nutritionist or even a health food enthusiast. A genius marketing idea, yes; a horrible weight-loss and long-term diet solution for health, most certainly.

Most diet plans or miracle weight-loss pills were created with dollar signs in sight, not the health and overall well-being of the many people who need help. These are the same people that the creators of these diets know will fall victim to their unrelenting marketing ploys and false claims of success. The bottom line is that most people are uneducated consumers, and the only form of education we're receiving is from television ads, social media, and the internet. Well, it's online, so it must be true, right? All of us are uneducated consumers, most on a daily basis. I know I am. I have to take the salesman's word at the car dealership that a double-sided airbag deployment system (if that is even such a thing) is not only the best thing for me and my family but exists and is

---

[12] "Almost 500 Foods Contain The 'Yoga Mat' Compound. Should ...." 6 Mar. 2014, https://www.npr.org/sections/thesalt/2014/03/06/286886095/almost-500-foods-contain-the-yoga-mat-compound-should-we-care-keep. Accessed 4 March. 2017.

actually a safety feature of my car. Really, how would I know otherwise unless Jay Leno had a free afternoon to go car shopping with me?

Like Increases Like

Certain truisms in nature can be found as an underlying aspect to your diet; seeing that all humans are a microcosm of the greater macrocosm. Or as stated in the Kybalion, "As above so below, and as below, so above." What is meant by this...? Simple: like increases like and opposites balance. These concepts are true within the universe and they are true within the human body. When looking upon your diet and daily lifestyle, these concepts must play a critical role in its formation and creation. If you can grasp this concept, combined with what you've been introduced and learned formerly, then it is easy to see how we must view our diet and our lifestyle. Knowing your *dosha* and the qualities of your foods and environment moves your diet from a game of guesses and wants, to a systematic theory of nourishment and preparation. Selecting the right foods and cooking and preparing them in a way that brings balance to your specific nature is a powerful way to manage your health and well-being. Your diet and lifestyle, which is referred to as *ahara* in Ayurveda, is one of three pillars of health. Proper sleep and regulating our sexual lives are the last two. By understanding this, it is easy to see how important our diet becomes, and the word diet will no longer hold the same significance for you moving forward.

Building upon the concepts of the 5 universal elements (*panchamahabhutas*), the three *tridoshas*, the six tastes (*rasa*), keys and classifications of proper digestion (*agni*) and the seven tissues (*Dhatus*), we can now explore the importance of proper food combinations, as well as wholesome vs. unwholesome foods.

A very important decision in Ayurveda, and it is one that is far too often overlooked in our society, is the importance of what foods are being consumed together, or better yet, food compatibility. There are 10 main categories of incompatible foods that we will concern ourselves with in this work. A common mistake, and this is one that I was committing regularly for years, is combining any form of dairy with any fruits - especially melons. Food incompatibilities are normally based upon the following criteria:

1. Potency of the foods
2. Processing
3. Preparation
4. Quantity / dose
5. Area of body digestion occurs
6. Enzymes required to process the foods
7. Rates of digestion
8. Time of year & seasonality

The consumption of improper food combinations, especially continually consumption, will lead to a disturbance in your digestion or *agni*, thus leading to the formation and accumulation of *ama*. This will, of course, result in some sort of imbalance or a state of dis-ease. Here is a list of the more common:

1. Dairy and most fruits, especially melons & banana
2. Fish and dairy
3. Milk and breads containing yeast
4. Honey and Ghee - note: never cook or heat honey over stove or flame
5. Grains with fruit and tapioca
6. Radishes with bananas, raisins and milk
7. Beanas with fruit, cheese, eggs, fish, milk, and yogurt
8. Lemon with milk, tomatoes and yogurt
9. Eggs with fruit, especially melons; beans, cheese, fish, kitchari, milk, meat, and yogurt
10. Yogurt with any of the following; fruit, cheese, eggs, fish, meat, milk and nightshades

Do you see a theme from above...? Correct, fruit should only be eaten with other fruits. I always recommend fruit to be consumed as a snack to help get you from meal A to meal B. I always added fruit, yogurt and milk to my after workout protein shakes. Today, though I still use various fruits in my smoothies, I've switched to an organic coconut milk and skip adding yogurt and/or cottage cheese. Those, like fruit, I typically consume alone as an in between meal snacks, especially in the warmer summer months. Immediately upon making the easy correction, I started noticing far less digestive disturbances, like excess gas or bloating. By paying attention to how my body was reacting I was successfully able to eliminate the root cause of, what most would look upon, as nagging discomfort or a funny amongst the guys.

Wholesome vs. Unwholesome Foods

The concept of wholesome foods in Ayurveda is based solely upon nourishing the body, pacifying of the *doshas* and the body's ability to digest and properly assimilate and eliminate the foods. Any food that does not fulfill the above is considered to be unwholesome or even junk food. I had a hard time at first wrapping my head around this particular concept. I remember saying to myself, "a carrot... how the hell can a carrot be considered junk food"? You see, the distinguishing factor here is three-fold: is this food compatible with my body-type (*prakriti* & *vikriti*), can I properly digest, assimilate & eliminate the food and does it aid in the generation and regeneration of tissue and other physiological matter? If the answer to any of those questions is no, then this food can and should be looked upon as unwholesome. There are, of course, varying degrees of this theory which I will leave for a later work.

Food: Energy & Vitality

As mentioned in the chapter entitled "The Five Elements," all foods are comprised of the five basic elements: space, air, fire, water and earth. These universal elements are also inherent in the fundamental creation of all matter, existing on the quantum level as fluxuations of certain energetic factors. Your specific body-type (*dosha*) is even a biological derivative of the energetic aspects of these elements. The relationship and formation of our bodily tissues can be linked to the elemental and energetic aspects of the foods that you consume.

The basic nature of our foods are consistent with their qualities, their tastes, as well as their nutritional attributes to the creation and formation of our bodies and our specific constitutional makeup. For instance, if it's cold outside and you're experiencing coldness internally, is it a good idea to consume something that is cold in temperature? No, I would hope you wouldn't. Ayurveda, however, takes this a step further in that you would not want to consume foods whose effect upon your body will only further exacerbate the quality of coldness. An example of this would be dairy, mint, or even cilantro. Healthy, yes. Not cold in their physical temperature, correct. They are, however, and this is the key to understanding this system, their attributes and pre and post digestive effect on the body is cooling in nature. It becomes important then to understand the qualities of the foods you consume and their physical and energetic effect on your body and your mind.

The main goal of your new diet will be based upon its ability to fit the above mold, or in Ayurvedic terms, we need to create a *sattwika* diet. This simply means a diet that is easy to digest and leaves very little residue after digestion (*ama*). This will leave the body feeling light and energetic, allowing for the flow of energy along their respective pathways (*srotas*) or meridians. A diet embodying *sattwika* will properly nourish all the tissues and vital organs alike, while keeping the mind and body in a compatible union.

There are four key concepts or principles which will not only properly assist in the balancing of the *dosha* and proper nourishment of bodily tissues and organs, but will also leave you in a state of energy and bliss. The four key components are as follows:

1. *Agni* - the energetic aspect of this metabolic fire provides energy to both the body and the mind - on the subtle and gross levels.
2. *Ojas* - the energetic essence of the *kapha dosha* that represents all the seven tissues (*dhatu*); it is the source of vitality, strength and immunity for the physical body.
3. *Tejas* - the energetic force that transforms matter into energy. It is an aspect of the *pitta dosha*.
4. *Prana* - the underlying energetic essence of all. This can be referred or likened to "Chi". This life force is the vital breath that animates and supports life. It is a very subtle essence of the *vata dosha*.

Understanding Prana

There is always an importance of understanding the nature upon which all creation is birthed into physical manifestation. By understanding the concept of *Prana* in Ayurveda, you will then begin to understand it as a caustitve force. All of the foods you consume and even the water you drink inherently contains *prana*. Looking at the foods you consume through the lens of this philosophy, you can now consider that everything you consume provides your body with the vital breath of life. It is of no surprise that the channels upon which *prana* is carried throughout the human body are rooted within the heart. When you overcook, freeze or microwave food, you are killing this vital energetic force that lives inherently within all living food, thus rendering the food dead. This is one of the main reasons why it is recommended to consume a certain percentage of raw or lightly steamed or sauteed foods. By doing so you are preserving this vital essence, which then gets transmuted into our bodies.

As you begin to see and understand now, the way you'll need to approach food and your diet is quite different from how you were formerly experiencing them. This will, of course, take some time to become familiar and comfortable, but just as in the formation of bad habits, we will persist together until this way of thinking becomes your new way of life. It is simple neuroplasticity, and together we will create the new neural connections that will pave a new way of thinking in the months and years to come.

The Eight Principles of Food

In the Ayurvedic model of food, there are eight governing principles which each of us must consider when creating any dietary program. The emphasis lies on the material and energetic qualities of food. The eight governing principles as laid forth in the *Charaka Samhita* are as follows[13]:

---

[13] "A glimpse of Ayurveda The forgotten history and ... - NCBI - NIH." 28 Feb. 2016, https://www.ncbi.nlm.nih.gov/pmc/articles/PMC5198827/. Accessed 14 Match. 2017.

1. Nature or Qualities of the Food
2. Preparation
3. Combination
4. Quantity
5. Habit and Climate
6. Time Factor
7. Rules of Use
8. The Consumer

There is an interesting aspect of food consumption to the Ayurvedic model. This is something which I often refer to as "compartmental eating". Meaning that it is stated in the treatise that the stomach capacity should be looked upon and divided into three parts; one part for solid foods, one part for water or other suitable liquids, and one part air. Leaving space for air is crucial in increasing your digestive fire. What is one of the elements needed to fuel your campfires... air!

During the process of eating, there are two additional factors that need to be consciously considered; small amounts of water consumed increases your digestive strength, while consuming larger amounts of water before, during or after the meal diminishes your digestive capacity. It clearly states in ancient texts of Ayurveda, the overconsumption of water after food is consumed leads to obesity. It must be understood that the foods you consume undergo a specific process of absorption, assimilation and transformation from physical matter into usable energetic substance by the body. This specific process fuels and generates all physiological functions. Each food is looked upon for its ability to be properly digested, and as mentioned above, if you cannot fully digest any particular food, then you need to view it as unwholesome.

Your body is a specific result of the foods you consume. There are four forms of consumables which we need to concern ourselves for the purpose of this work - they are as follows:

1. Eatables
2. Liquid, drinkables
3. Linctus (liquidy and gooey deliverables, usually used in transportation of medicinals)
4. Masticable foods

When looking at the principles of food according to Ayurveda, it appears that consuming foods that are properly prepared to ensure maximum digestion is a key factor. Consuming foods that have been slightly cooked and are unctuous in nature, in general, sets the stage for the highest level of digestibility. When properly prepared, the foods you consume will heighten your digestive fire, carminates gas, becomes easily absorbed, increases strength and produces a light and energetic sensation. Oh... and I forgot to mention - they'll taste better. This process promotes life and mental clarity, as well as keeps the precise equilibrium of the *tridoshas*.

While consuming your meals there are a few aspects that I want you to become mindful of:

1. Don't eat too fast or too slow
2. Fully masticate your foods
3. Do not eat meals when upset
4. Become mindful in the act of eating

Here is the reality of this philosophy; these are easy acts to perform as well as incorporate into your daily routine. If you are truly needing or wanting to live a balanced life, then following and mastering these essential principles should become your focus moving forward. These are actions I expect of myself. You, too, should be the wiser.

Mind, The Psychosomatic Effect

"The body and the mind are the abodes of diseases as well as health. Proper body-mind interaction is the cause for happiness."
- **Charaka Samhita, Chapter 1, verse 55**

थे बोद्य् अन्द् थे मिन्द् अरे अबोदेस ओफ़ दिसेअसेस् अस वेल्ल अस हेअल्थ्:
प्रोपेर बोद्य्-मिन्द् मेदिचिने इस थे चौसे ओफ़ हप्पिनेस्स

**shareer aur man rogon ke saath-saath svaasthy ka nivaas hai.
uchit shareer-man antahkaran sukh ka kaaran hai.**

If you walked down any street in suburbia America 50 years ago around 5 o'clock in the evening, you would've bore witness to families sitting around the dinner table sharing a meal with a smile upon their faces. Take a stroll down those streets today, however, and you'll come to notice something entirely different; empty tables and the faces of the many buried into some sort of electronic device. Sharing a meal with your family has become, of course, not for all, a long lost tradition. The figures supporting this realization are astounding. According to Forbes, over half of Americans either eat alone, at restaurants, at work or on the go. This is largely due to our fast-paced - always on the go society, as well as given the fact that we've become a society of snackaholics. I was startled, to say the least. You must ask yourself, why is sitting down at the dinner table important?

The irony of the situation, however, lies within the reasoning behind its importance. Holding strong to the differences between the conventional approach to health and the Ayurvedic standpoint, the important things are still quite unique. Falling under the conventional approach you'll come to understand that sharing a meal with your family creates a stronger family bond and instills greater family interaction. Those are, of course, positive and important reasons to share meals together with family and friends. The Ayurvedic outlook, though similar in the above reasoning, takes a much more comprehensive approach. This approach is centered around one of the most important fundamentals of Ayurveda, digestion.

The importance of this theory has far more to do with the person's frame of mind than it does ensuring that mommy and daddy are seated next to you. One of the most important aspects of nutrition is the mental and emotional state of the consumer. The influence of negative emotions, meaning residing in the wrong state of mind, thwarts the digestive process more than consuming incompatible foods or even foods that are aggravating for your *doshic* makeup. Healthy and wholesome foods, even when consumed in states of anger, fear, greed, just to name a few, cannot be digested properly. I repeat... ARE NOT properly digested. The effects can be severely detrimental to your health and overall well-being. This philosophy reflects the following: humans are emotional creatures and the body and mind connection is the unseen governing force behind our true state of health. Dr. Vasant Lad, the foremost expert on Ayurveda here in the US, is quoted saying "emotions are like mangos. We have to learn to ripen them and then juice them. When emotions are juiced, they are deeply nourishing and sweet [14].

---

[14] "The Link Between Your Emotions and Your Digestion | The ...." 8 Jul. 2015, https://chopra.com/articles/the-link-between-your-emotions-and-your-digestion. Accessed 14 Mar. 2017.

Mindful vs. Mindless Eating

So, what is the key to ensuring that you're going to be able to effectively digest your meals? Simple: be mindful! When you're consuming food it is crucial to focus on the art or act of eating. What does this mean? First before I answer this question, here is the short list of characteristics for something I like to call, mindless eating:

1. Overeating
2. Emotional eating
3. Eating on the go
4. Eating at random and sporadic times
5. Eating & multi-tasking
6. Rapid or fast eating

Let's take a moment and look at the aspects of mindless eating and its negative impact on your state of health. Take for instance, number six above. When you consume your food quickly you are not allowing for the establishment of the crucial communication between the body and brain. By eating quickly, you will often times end up consuming too much food before your brain receives the information which in turn sends a signal for you to stop eating. The information coming from the body to the brain can take 20 minutes. If you are eating rapidly and mindlessly you will surely consume far more than you need to properly nourish the body and feel satiated. The result: an over consumption of food.

I consider mindless eating to be an ever-growing epidemic in the U.S. Not understanding or not being fully aware of your body's hunger signals is another common example of mindless eating. Not understanding how to properly interpret or fully understand the language your body speaks can lead to various digestional and health-related disturbances. Do not reside only within the realm of your conscious intellect. Reach down and look within and establish a strong line of communication with your body. Doing so will help to ensure that you are not overeating or eating for emotional reasons. Remember, the one true goal of food consumption is to nourish the body and to support life; not for social or emotional reasons.

Another characteristic of mindless eating is probably what you've become most accustomed to referring to as "random eating". Do you often find yourself rummage around the fridge or cupboards at random times for no particular reason, other than perhaps boredom? This strongly indicates that you could be unknowingly participating in mindless eating.

Social eating is in my opinion one of the more common agents driving your mindless eating. Social eating encompasses a wide range of characteristics. One being, of course, trying to keep up with the Jones, so to speak. I often fall victim to this aspect of mindless eating. When you find yourself in a social setting where there is an abundance of unhealthy food options, it does in fact become difficult not to join your friends in this very common form of social interaction. All of those glorious wings, the pizza oozing with melted cheese, the salty abundance of fries, and of course... we cannot forget the booze! Is you mouth watering? Are you starting to feel hungry? If so, then we need to look at this aspect of mindless eating later in the customized version of this work.

The next characteristic of mindless eating is commonly found in those who are overweight or those suffering from obesity. One important distinction in mindless eating is what is known more commonly as emotional eating. Ask yourself, are you reaching for foods which are satisfying your emotions or foods that are properly supporting the health of your mind and body? Usually with this aspect of mindless eating there are underlying psychological or deeply ceded subconscious factors which need to be first addressed and corrected. I am sure you are consciously aware of the fact that the gallon of ice cream you scoffed down last night while watching an emotionally purging movie was not the best choice. The need to satisfy the emotional aspect of your desires is stemming from the depth of your subconscious mind. It is here where you will need to literally unlearn and relearn new behaviors. Hypnosis, in my opinion, is one of the more effective modalities when confronted with emotional and psychological undertones.

A very important consideration which has become an important component of our diets according to Ayurveda, is the life cycle of the food. We must ask ourselves, where did this food come from? Where, how and what time of year was this food harvested? All of these considerations do in fact affect the state of your body's ability to properly digest them, as well as their effect on your *dosha*. Most of us today have lost our connection to our foods. This is not only disappointing, but this is far removed from our hunter and gatherer ancestors. All is one and one is all. Understanding the true meaning behind this will afford you the wisdom to comprehend the importance of establishing a connection with the food we consume. Grace and giving thanks is also an aspect of this in which we will look at further in this work. With that said, let's look at the ever important aspects of "mindful" eating. I consider the following to be the more important facets in which best fits the Ayurvedic model:

- Fully chew your foods
- Listen to your body, stop just before feeling full
- Eat at specific times & places in correlation with your specific *dosha*
- Consume wholesome foods that supports your specific make-up
- Only eat when eating
- Ask, "Am I going to be able to digest this...?"
- Eat to support life, not your emotions

As you can see, mindfulness or "mindful eating" means residing in the present moment. When consuming your meals, focus on the act of eating. It is a skill... an art that must be correctly performed. Do not watch TV or movies, especially of a scary or thrilling nature. Do not perform work duties while eating, and never - never eat when upset or angry. Accept the joyous nature of eating, bask in the moment and connect with your foods.

The above suggestions, like most of the Ayurvedic model, is not difficult to understand nor should they present you any challenges when trying to ingrain them into your new regimen. Take fully masticating your food. This is a basic skill which not only have we forgotten, but sadly most of us were never properly taught. Sure it is an easy act to perform, but it is a learned skill - as all of the above are learned and adopted behaviors. By fully chewing your foods this automatically will allow you to eat slower and more methodically, thus giving the much needed communication between your brain and body to occur. By stopping slightly before feeling full, you will give your brain the last few minutes it needs to ultimately determine that you are in fact full. You can now walk away feeling properly satiated and energetic, rather than feeling stuffed, bloated and tired.

There is a universal principle hidden away within the realm of the quantum world that plays a role in the inefficacy or efficacy of mindful eating habits. The act of eating, as all in the universe, falls under the law of cause and effect. What do I mean by this? Allow me to use a hypothetical example to explain this for you.

Let's look at not properly chewing your food as an example to help illustrate my point. For the sake of this argument, assume for a moment that you are someone who swallows their food with the least amount of chews possible. I think we've all been guilty of this at least a few times during our lives. The result or effect of this can be quite profound: by ineffectively chewing your food, you are in fact also eating quickly. By consuming your meal quickly you're not allowing the appropriate amount of time for the brain and body to communicate. This is done via the hormone, ghrelin, and it's an essential fundamental biological process. The brain eventually receives the notice that you are in fact full, however, it's too late - once again you've overeaten. In addition, not only has the lining of your stomach now stretched to accommodate the excess food, this over-abundance of food is only partially masticated.

You now starting to feel sluggish, but resting is not an option for you considering that you are at work and your boss is screaming due to the fact that you failed to meet your sales quota for the week. Sensing his anger, this abruptly forces you into fight or flight mode where the only active area of your brain is the amygdala. The hostility being expressed from your boss tells your brain to secrete adrenaline and cortisol, amongst a slew of other hormones. Now, all of the blood that was being fed to your stomach in order to aid in digestion, is now being redirected and pumped to your limbs. Why...? Your brain is perceiving danger and immediately prepares for a physical altercation or the need to run. The rapid secretion of hormones instantly warms-up your body as to prevent injury if in fact you do have fight or high-tail it out of there.

Several minutes later your conscious mind regains control of the situation and overrides the primitive aspects of your mind and tells the body that you are no longer in danger. Although you are no longer in any physical danger, given the fact that you cannot release the stress caused by the event, you are still residing in a heightened emotional state. You are consciously aware that you cannot walk up to your boss and punch him square in his nose at this moment, so to help you deal with the stress you head to the snack machine to grab a Pop Tarts and of course, a sugary cup-o-coffee. You quickly consume them both, only momentarily feeling better. You then resume to make your sales calls. At this point, the partially chewed food-stuff from your lunch is still undigested in your stomach, on top of which you've now added more indigestible food. This begins to cause minor, and what you've always considered, annoying digestive disturbances. Now, since this is not the first time this scenario has happened, your digestional tract also houses bezoars, which are hardened bits of food matter caused by foodstuff that was left undigested in your stomach. These bezoars are the result of similar experiences which happened earlier in the year. You now find yourself in a pretty serious state - a state which could've been easily avoided if you were a mindful eater instead of a mindless eater. So, you see, every action, every decision faithfully obeys the laws of cause and effect. The above scenario illustrates that three minor acts of mindless eating, not fully chewing your food, eating too rapidly and eating while in a state of stress, is the root cause of a fairly serious imbalance. Even in this diegesis, one cannot escape the grips of the law of cause and effect. It happens all the time and is unrelenting in its course.

The last few aspects pertaining to mindful eating will be determined once we properly assess the state of your *dosha*. This will tell us the times of day you'll want to consume your meals, as well as what foods best fits your unique and specific situation. Add those to the latter and we've just established a very strong nutritional foundation for you moving forward. We will, of course, get more specific and tweak this along the way, but let's move on with the mind and its relationship upon your digestion.

The PathWay of the Mind

The Ayurvedic model takes into account the relationship the mind plays when determining the overall health of a person and in treating certain aspects of disease. The slightest disturbance in the mind can affect many physiological systems and pathways, thus resulting in a disorder of the *doshas*. Since the mind plays such an important role in your health, Ayurveda has passed forth many effective modalities to help ensure a balanced relationship exists between our minds and bodies.

Energetic substances move accordingly throughout the body via various and distinct channels. As I mentioned prior, the mind has its own channel for the movement of this energetic substance. In Sanskrit it is referred to as *mano vaha srotas*. One very important aspect to understand is the location of the mind within the human body. Most here in the West, if asked, would assume that the mind resides in the brain. It does not, and this is the exact premise of the Ayurvedic model. The seat of the mind or the root of the mind in the body, according to Ayurveda, does not exist in the brain... but rather in the heart. Yes, the heart is the root area of the body where the mind originates from, however, mind is present and encompasses the whole being holographically. All of the Vedic sciences, which includes Ayurveda and Yoga, view the significance of the heart in our overall balance and well-being. Of the thirteen pathways within the human body (*srotas*), three of these pathways originate in the heart.

Is this timeless philosophical distinction of Ayurveda matching what the latest scientific discoveries of our time is now telling us? It has been mapped that the auric field emanating from the heart extends farther into the ether than it does anywhere else. This bio-field is energetic in its nature, electromagnetic to be precise. This points us to discern that the strongest area of electrical impulses coming from our bodies does not in fact emanate from the brain, they come from our hearts. These subtle bio-fields are generated by all living cells, tissues and organs. Why...? Simple: we are nothing other than energetic beings. Keeping this in mind, can you recall earlier when I was describing the aspects of the 5 universal elements to be energetic in nature and that we need to view them not as the physically manifest matter of water and fire and earth, but rather the subtler aspects of their nature?

The concept of morphogenetic fields, first discovered by Rupert Sheldrake, very closely mirrors the concept of mind and its relationship to the human body. Within this energy field exist what he referred to as a "morphic unit"[15]. These morphic units are the developmental aspects of tissue. As an example, the cardiac field is responsible for the creation of the tissue making up your heart. Through resonance all tissue within the human body is constructed.

---

[15] "Scientific Heretic Rupert Sheldrake on Morphic Fields, Psychic ...." 14 Jul. 2014, https://blogs.scientificamerican.com/cross-check/scientific-heretic-rupert-sheldrake-on-morphic-fields-psychic-dogs-and-other-mysteries/. Accessed 25 March. 2017.

Mind is the glue linking the field through resonance to our bodies. From the Ayurvedic viewpoint, the subtle channels (*nadis*) are believed to carry the flow of *prana* from the base of the spine to the crown of the head. These specific locations are, of course, the chakra centers of the body. The flow of *prana* along these pathways establishes the innate relationship between our minds, hearts and God.

We now understand that the heart is the root center in the human body for the mind. Interestingly, however, the pathways for mind exist throughout the entire body *mano vaha srotas*[16]. By influencing the entire body, the vast encompassing power of this pathway makes it the most profound aspect when we look at establishing balance or fighting disease. There is a very important distinction here, however, that you must grasp before moving on; the mind affects all areas of the body, as well as those areas that can equally affect the mind. This process is a two-way street, though, in my opinion, the mind affecting the body is a greater causative factor. These inner highways or pathways are responsible for the transportation of divergent functions, both subtle and gross, as well as energetic and biological. These channels are completely distinct from our veins and other gross pathways located within the human body, so the two are not to be confused. When looking through the lens of this model, each cell that comprises the human body can be looked upon as a *srotas*. Each of our cells is in constant communication with the etheric field encompassing its being. The communication is also a dual

---

[16] "Nourishing Manovaha Srotas | Banyan Botanicals." 25 Oct. 2012, https://www.banyanbotanicals.com/info/blog-banyan-vine/details/nourishing-manovaha-srotas/. Accessed 25 March. 2017.

channel, and information is constantly being sent and received. There are, of course, just like any highway system, doors and exits located throughout the various pathways. These openings or doorways play a crucial role in the maintenance of the pathways. They influence each respected channel and they are often used as an opening to help restore balance to any disturbed area or channel.

You should be well aware by now that an impaired digestive state results in the formation of toxic *ama*, and interestingly enough, the mind is no exception to this rule. Unresolved emotions and other various mental imbalances leads to a mental aspect of *ama*, which in turn is one of the main causative factors in the disease process. For example, unresolved anger can accumulate in the liver and impair its functioning. Unprocessed grief can disturb the lungs, and chronic anxiety can upset the health of the colon[17]. Knowing how the mind can affect these various biological systems and organs becomes an ever important aspect in the pathogenic aspect of disease detection and elimination.

The importance that the mind plays on the overall health of our bodies and their vast pathways and functioning is something that I cannot stress enough. The philosophical aspects of the mind and its effect on the body is another principle that is bound by the law of cause and effect. Think negative or destructive thoughts and you'll experience negative emotions. Holding onto and residing from a heightened state of negative emotions leads to the

---

[17] David Frawley, *Ayurveda and the Mind: The Healing of Consciousness* (Lotus Press, 1997) p. 103

formation of mental *ama*. This form of *ama*, as you've been just introduced to, leads to disturbances and imbalances in a number of relative systems and biological functions. It is for precisely these reasons why a large aspect of the Ayurvedic model focuses on the cultivation, prevention and correction of mental imbalances as a first step. Yoga and mediation are two very effective modalities that were created within the scope of the Vedic model in order to help ensure that a state of balance exists in our psycho-spiritual and biological health.

Qualities of Consciousness, the Universal Attributes

The term quality or attribute in Ayurveda is called, *guna*. So the quality or *guna* of the mind is referred to as *maha guna*, or quality of the mind. There is nothing in existence that does not possess the subtle nature of the three aspects of *maha guna*. The three subtle qualities in Ayurveda are; *sattva*, *rajas*, and *tamas*[18]. The subtle qualities of *sattva*, *rajas*, and *tamas* are delicately interwoven throughout the fabric of life. Each aspect represents certain distinct characteristics. Here is a breakdown of the unique qualities of the three *maha gunas*:

1. **Sattva** - this is the *guna* of clarity. It represents purity, intelligence and light. This guna is responsible for the perception of wisdom from the cosmic intelligent field, and represents a clear knowledge.

---

[18] "Vedic Yoga and the Three Gunas - Yoga Veda Institute."
https://www.yogavedainstitute.com/wp-content/uploads/2016/01/The_Three_Gunas_PDF.pdf.
Accessed 7 Jan. 2018.

2. **Rajas** - this is the *guna* responsible for activity, or energetic aspects of change and transformation. It is represented by passion, but also agitation. It is the movement of light from the darkness set forth by *tamas*.
3. **Tamas** - this is the *guna* responsible for interia. Its nature is that of sleep, dullness, lethargy and often times negativity. It is within the darkness of *tamas* that solidity is manifested, just as how the creation of matter happened after the explosion of the Big Bang.

The delicate interweaving of the energetic aspects of the three *gunas* in our lives are always present and are working in unison with the ebb and flow of creation. With that said, however, the Vedic Scriptures point us towards an affinity for *sattva guna*, mainly due to its direct relationship to the process of inner enlightenment. Just as in a recipe for apple pie, add more brown sugar and the end result will be that much more sweeter and appealing to the palate. Imbalances can also be directly related to disturbances within any area of the three universal qualities. This is a very systematic approach in uncovering the pathogenic factors contributing to any disturbances or imbalances. To respect the brilliance of this system and its simplicity of use is to understand the processes of human creation. And as we proceed even further in this work, you'll come to appreciate and understand this even more.

Mental Constitution

The science of Ayurveda is an awesome organization of cause and effect that is intermingled throughout the fabric of our bodies and their relationship to the Universe. Our mental constitution or makeup, which is called *manas prakriti* in Ayurveda, is similar and uniquely marries that of our *dosha*. Their similarities are abundant, however, there is one very distinct aspect that you need to understand. Unlike your *prakriti* or doshic makeup that was set forth at the time of your conception, your mental makeup can and often changes throughout your lifetime. It is a tempermental dance upon the backdrop of your *doshic* foundation which is continually creating the current state of your *dosha* (*vikriti*). As you evolve in consciousness, the state of your *manas prakriti* is affected positively. This resembles many other traditional forms of holistic arts. The state of your *manas prakriti* does relate to the state of your *dosha*, however, the state of your *doshic*-makeup also affects the state of your mental constitution (*manas prakriti*). Life is a continual swing of the pendulum, ranging from one side to another, being controlled by the mind and its relationship to the body and to the Universe.

Each of the *tridoshas* has its corresponding mental component; the *vata* mind, pitta *and* the *kapha* mind. It is important to note that the constitution of the mind does not have to match that of the primary *dosha* of the individual. Oftentimes, they are not the same. As an example, my physiological makeup is primarily *pitta*, though I possess higher qualities of the *vata* mind. Let's take a more in depth look into the three variations.

The Vata Mind

They are referred to as quick witty, active, moves fast and talks even faster. They possess qualities of the elemental factors of the *vata dosha*. The elemental forces responsible for the creation of the *vata dosha* will also be the factors inherent within the characteristics of the mind. In keeping with the example at the start of this section, the imbalanced *vata* mind is anxious, over sensitive and often times very unstable. Those manifestations all resemble the unique characteristics of the space and air elements. The law of polarity, which states that everything in the universe is merely one side of its opposing nature, (hot & cold), is at play when we look at the relationship of the body to the mind. In the body, when the *vata dosha* is out of alignment it can cause a multitude of manifestations in your behavior, such as anxiety, nervousness, lack of direction, fear and a general sensation of not being grounded.

When the mind is out of balance but not as a direct result of a disturbance in the *dosha*, it is usually from social behaviors such as being overworked, stressed, or frequent acts of multitasking. Any of these behaviors are often the culprit for the vitiation of the *vata* mind. And knowing that all of life is a play of cause and effect, an aggravation of the *vata* mind can lead to an imbalance in the *dosha* - around and around we go. Even exposure to frequent loud music and an overconsumption of stimulants like cigarettes and caffeine can also cause a vitiation of the mind. The *vata* mind correlates to the *sattva guna*.

The Pitta Mind

The *pitta* mind can oftentimes be the hardest of the three aspects of mind to assess. It is not as thorough and nonchalaunt as the *kapha* mind, but it is not an erratic and ever-changing as its *vata* counterpart. It is formed from the fire and water elements, and it is responsible for the governing of the intellect and for the transformation of stimuli from the external world. It closely relates to the gray matter of the brain and is very closely intertwined with the *rajasic* nature of the mind. Displays of confidence and enthusiasm are tell-tale signs for the robust nature of the *pitta* mind.

When out of balance, the *pitta* mind can result in anger and hostility on the one end, and irritability and resentment on the other end. Someone displaying an over-critical nature and someone who is too ambitious often leads us to believe there is a vitiation of the *pitta* mind. Excess heat moving upward in the body is also an underlying cause of excess *pitta* in the mind.

The Kapha Mind

The white matter, adipose tissue and the nervous tissue of the brain are directly related in nature to the *kapha* mind. Being formed from the water and earth elements, the *kapha* mind is associated with our memories. The *kapha* mind is also closely related to *tamasic* qualities. The slow moving and dark aspects of the *kapha* mind can result in attachment and depression. When balanced, however, it can signal love, stability, compassion and groundedness.

An accumulation of the water and earth elements in the mind can lead to aggravation of the *kapha* mind. An unbalanced *kapha* mind has a tendency to display lethargy, stubbornness, depression and an increase of emotional possessiveness. This last manifestation, however, is tricky. The *kapha* type even when balanced is very loyal and demonstrates a unique level of allegiancy. The overall goal for a person of the *kapha* nature is essentially to get moving! The flip side of that coin, however, can lead to an increase of the water and earth elements in the mind causing a vitiation of the *kapha* mind. Proper exercise and consuming foods higher in the bitter and pungent tastes also helps in pacifying the heaviness of earth and water, thus alleviating the excess of these elements within the mind.

The key for living in a balanced state is to understand that more often than not the mind is the root cause of whatever illness you may currently be suffering. If this is in fact the case, it is in the mind where the imbalance or correction must first occur. This will produce effective and efficient results, thus positively affecting the body. Hypnosis and its many amazing branches may offer scientific proof to the efficacy of how important and influential the mind can be when governing our physical bodies as well as our overall state of health.

Eat Your Medicine

"Even an acute poison can become an excellent drug if it is properly administered. On the other hand even a drug, if not properly administered, becomes an acute poison."
- Charaka sutra sthana, Chapter 24, verse 126

योगादपिविषंतीक्ष्णमुत्तमं भेषजं भवेत्|

भेषजं चापि दुर्युक्तं तीक्ष्णं सम्पद्यते विषय||१२६||

Yogaadapi visham tikshmuttam bheshajam bhavet, bheshjam chaapi duryuktam tiksham sampadhyate visham

I've come to realize that the above quote may seem strange, especially given the fact that today's foods and medicines are making us sicker than we've ever been. The majority of what we eat as a modernized society should no longer be called food. It should be relabeled as "food-like" substance. Our foods today are nutritionally devoid of the essential vitamins and minerals that we as humans need to survive, leaving most Americans starving on a nutritional level. This is a paradox of sorts: we are starving nutritionally, however, most are insatiable when it comes to the consumption of sugars, fats and salts. One major goal in writing this book for you is to bring light to the importance of this subject and at the same time provide the knowledge, motivation and means for you to easily incorporate them into your life.

Many today are aware that Hippocrates was the founder of what's considered modern-day medicine. Hence, this is where the term "hippocratic oath" is derived from. Of those who are aware of this, most are unaware that he was also one of the first to realize that disease was not caused by an angry or vengeful God[19]. He understood that the process of disease lived in the humoral theory - the exact same theory that I've written this book upon. Hippocrates and the followers of his time believed and supported the theory that all disease arises out of an imbalance of the bodily humors. The only difference from his philosophy and that of the Ayurvedic model, is that he suggested that there are four bodily humors, not three as suggested by Ayurveda.

Viewing food as medicine is complex and has many varying degrees leading to countless theories and interpretations. The Ayurvedic model of medicine, for one, is a strong voice for the validity of looking upon our foods as medicine. It is only when improper foods are improperly consumed is when the need for medical intervention is often needed. Hippocrates and other Hippocratic trained physicians of his time, however, clearly saw a difference between food and pharmaceutical medicines. In fact, food was considered as a material that could be assimilated by the human body after digestion occurred. Other elements such as air and the sun were also considered food due to the fact the body was able to convert them into the various substances of the body. As an example, food is converted into the different parts of the body such as muscles, tissues and nerves, just to name a few. By contrast, the concept of

---

[19] "Health care practices in ancient Greece: The ... - NCBI." 15 Mar. 2014, https://www.ncbi.nlm.nih.gov/pmc/articles/PMC4263393/. Accessed 9 March. 2018.

medicine at this time was a product which was able to change the body's own nature (in terms of humor quality or quantity) but could not be converted into the body's own substance. Thus, to Hippocrates, food wasn't considered a medicine[20]. The Ayurvedic models disagrees.

The six tastes are one of the more important factors stressed by Ayurveda when looking upon our food as medicine. Ayurveda considers the taste, the quality and the pre and post-digestive effect on the body as the karmic efficacy that the food or drug has on the body. A well-balanced diet, meaning a diet that incorporates the appropriate amounts of the six tastes in relation to that person's specific *dosha* will maintain the proper state of homeostasis. Sadly, the opposite is also true. Looking upon food as medicine within the Ayurvedic realm exists as a system of balance and of like increases like. When we consume a balanced array of wholesome foods, prepared and consumed in the correct fashion and within the proper state of mind, then man-made pharmaceuticals become of no use. This reminds me of an ancient Ayurvedic proverb, "When diet is wrong, medicine is of no use. When diet is correct, medicine is of no need.[21]"

The Ayurvedic model of medicine, which is the oldest form of organized medicine still in use today, is built upon the premise that it is better to avoid than fix - prevent rather than cure. Simply employ the force of its opposite nature to reduce excess or lack. This foundation is supported through various

---

[20] "Let food be thy medicine… - NCBI." https://www.ncbi.nlm.nih.gov/pmc/articles/PMC318470/. Accessed 9 March. 2018.
[21] "Ayurveda - Wikiquote." https://en.wikiquote.org/wiki/Ayurveda. Accessed 9 March. 2018.

modalities within the scope of Ayurveda and treating our foods as a main source of medicine is surely one of them. As an example, let's take the case of a fever. This is the result of an increase of the *pitta dosha*, therefore, herbs and foods of a cooling and bitter nature will need to be used to decrease the excess heat caused by the fire element. Conventional or modern medicine does not recognize pharmacological attributes to the six tastes. Only in the last decade has there been promising studies showing the possibility of a correlation between taste and pharmacology. I find it amazing that it has taken modern science over 5,000 years to just begin to recognize something that is the foundation of a science created so many decades ago. It has also been recently discovered that specific combinations of the six tastes (*rasa*) in Ayurveda correlates with specific enzyme active sites in the body[22]. It is at the subtle energetic level that modern-day scientists will soon be able to link the six tastes with curative distinctions in the human body, especially since the government says that the drastic rise of healthcare cost is a major concern for this country moving forward. I guess, perhaps, only time will tell. For now, let's only concern ourselves with the Ayurvedic approach to healthcare. Here is an in-depth example of how the science of Ayurveda looks upon foods which we would only consider as cooking spices.

Common Name	Sanskrit Name	Taste	Qualities	Properties
Cumin	Jira	Bitter, pungent & Astringent	Increases P Pacifies V, K	Promotes Digestion

---

[22] "Exploring Ayurvedic Knowledge on Food and Health ... - NCBI." 31 Mar. 2016, https://www.ncbi.nlm.nih.gov/pmc/articles/PMC4815005/. Accessed 10 March. 2018.

Turmeric	Haldi	Bitter, pungent & Astringent	Increases V, P Pacifies K	Anti-inflammatory
Ginger	Adrakh	Pungent & Sweet	Increases P Pacifies V, K	Digestive Aid, Carminative
Black Pepper	Kali Mirch	Pungent	Increases P Pacifies V, K	Stimulant, Decongestant
Coriander	Dhania	Sweet, Astringent	Pacifies all doshas	Lowers Blood Sugars

The above are prime examples of how Ayurveda looks at foods and their effect and relationship to your overall well-being. In Part Two of this book we will look at more of the common foods you're consuming, as well as lay out their effect on your mind and your body.

When viewing food as medicine we need to concern ourselves with four additional and very important categories. Do the foods you're consuming adhere to the following:

1. Properly nourish
2. Detox
3. Control inflammation
4. Effect on the body's pH level

Let's discuss the above components.

Properly Nourish

Physiological and mental nourishment are the two key aspects of health and our well-being. The maintenance, reproduction and growth of our bodies and minds are governed through a process of gross and subtle nourishment. We learned earlier that the foods you consume are digested, assimilated and transformed into our bodily tissues and organs in a very specific manner. In addition, our foods are also processed into an energetic substance that is ultimately transmogrified into consciousness.

The process of cell generation and regeneration is a critical aspect to even the conventional approach to medicine. The conventional approach views cell growth in terms of cell population. Each population of cells, which directly corresponds to certain biochemical and bioenergetic processes, endures a growth process that is referred to as doubling. During this process, in theory, the population of the cells should double in their size. This, however, is not the case under most circumstances. Lack of proper nutritional components, as well as mental disturbances cause an undergrowth of the cells' population. In essence, your body's current liver is only as healthy and effective as the foods you ate approximately 45 days ago; 15 days for the food to be converted into the substance used in cell reproduction, and another 30 days for the cells of the liver, called hepatocytes, to regenerate into what is ultimately a newer version of your liver[23]. Over consumption of substances like Tylenol, creates a disturbance within the cellular health of the liver, however, through the above

---

[23] "Liver regeneration - Wikipedia." https://en.wikipedia.org/wiki/Liver_regeneration. Accessed 11 March. 2018.

process, the liver can heal itself within the given time frame. If you were, however, fueling your body via unhealthy foods devoid of the essential nutrients the cells of the liver requires, then the state of the liver will not be quite as effective as it once was - or as effective as it should be. As an example, vitamin K is essential in the protein production induced by the liver for blood clotting purposes[24]. The liver is one of the more important organs in the body with regards to this premise due to the fact that the liver is one of the main organs responsible for the conversion of the food we eat into substances that the body requires. Liver health and liver detoxification, which we will look at in greater detail in Part Two, is crucial when trying to maintain a balanced state of health.

The next aspect we need to consider when viewing proper nourishment, and it is of utmost importance within the view of Ayurveda, is the nourishment of the *doshas* and ultimately each of its subsequent systems. Ayurveda considers that we are merely a microcosm of the greater universal macrocosm. Your reality is a unique and intelligent layering of energetic information, so too is your body. It is constructed upon layers of energetic or concentric fields which overlap and work in unison with one another. When you look upon the human body through the lens of this truth, understanding the importance of proper nutrition becomes an essential factor that directly relates to what you see in the mirror each and every day.

---

[24] Schmidt R, Lang F, Heckmann M. Physiologie des Menschen: mit Pathophysiologie. Heidelberg: Springer; 2011.

Each of the *tridoshas* have *subdosha*s which are directly related to the process of properly nourishing the tissues, organs and systems of the body. As an example, one of the *subdosha*s of *pitta* that is responsible for the spleen, liver and blood is referred to as *ranjaka pitta*. It is this aspect of the *pitta dosha* that is responsible for the dominion over the skin and disturbances such as discolorations, cirrhosis, high cholesterol, hepatitis, chronic fatigue syndrome, emotional overload and blood issues[25]. The red blood cells of our body are directly related to this process, but if we are not consuming foods which are vital in the production of red blood cells like beans, legumes and organic egg yolks, the *ranjaka pitta* will become vitiated. If left uncorrected, a disturbance of this *subdosha* might ultimately result as a manifestation of some sort of skin condition. Taking this even a step further, the western approach would more times than not prescribe some sort of topical pharmaceutical intervention, that though may provide temporary relief of the manifested symptom, will never correct the root cause of the imbalance.

I am not going to go into all 15 *subdoshas*, but I will go over two more profound examples supporting their importance. Once we assess your *dosha*, its specific state, as well as the state of your digestion and overall lifestyle, it will be more of a concern for myself to ensure that each of the 15 *subdoshas* are properly supporting the overall state of your *prakriti*. One of the more important *subdoshas* which you need to be concerned with is the *prana subdosha*, which falls under the *vata dosha*. The *prana subdosha* is responsible

---

[25] "Ayurvedic Sub-Doshas And How To Best Nourish Them ...." 11 Apr. 2017, https://basmati.com/2017/04/11/ayurvedic-sub-doshas-and-how-best-nourish-them. Accessed 11 March. 2018.

for the governing of the energetic life forces through which the body acquires through various foods and other subtler means. Foods that are consumed as close to their natural state will possess higher levels of *prana*. Various herbs and whole foods will help supply the body with this inherent form of consciousness. The *prana subdosha* is directly related to our nervous system, as well as responsible for maintaining a state of homeostasis. So, you see, when you consume an abundance of foods that are considered non-nourishing, such as chips, cookies and other highly processed treats, you are consuming food that is considered to be dead under the scope of the Ayurvedic model. The goal of your customized version of this work will be to not only incorporate whole and living foods into your diet, but make them appealing to your palate and other senses as well.

Each *dosha* has its 5 corresponding *subdoshas*, and though they are all important, one from each of the *tridoshas* stands out as the pinnacle of each of their respective *subdoshas*. The *subdoshas* of the *kapha dosha* that we will concern ourselves with in this section is called *avalambaka*. The *avalambaka* aspect of the *kapha dosha* governs the heart and the lungs. Pretty important... I think so! By being responsible for the overall dispersal of nourishment to the entire body, ensuring a balanced state of this *subdosha* is also something that we will concern ourselves with as we move forward in the creation of your specific lifestyle plan. As you should now be aware of, nourishment doesn't always happen through our foods. They happen via the air, sensory intake, as well as the mind. Practices such as Yoga Nidra and *pranayama* are excellent modalities which can help to balance and restore the *avalambak dosha* to its natural state. Therapies such as this will be specifically prescribed in the custom version of this book.

By becoming more aware of these and other subtler aspects of your body, it places you in a position where balancing and rebalancing becomes much easier and far less invasive. Oh, and did I mention, far less expensive! This relates to what I mentioned earlier in this work when I said that you must understand and become fluent in the language spoken by your body. By understanding the various ways through which nourishment occurs, you will become just that more fluent in the tongue of your body... and just that much more powerful.

Detoxification

I read somewhere that we as humans should regularly detox our bodies, our minds and our contacts lists. The importance of proper detoxification is crucial even under conditions when we could be considered to be residing in a healthy state. Can you imagine its significance in today's modern world?

If we knew what we were consuming most of the time, I am willing to bet we would not be unconsciously shoveling that extra cheesy bacon burrito so vehemently into our mouths. The disgusting fact is that I am not even talking about the plethora of loogies, hair, skin and other assorted goodies and bugs which fall into our foods on a daily basis. No, I am talking about the vast array of over 100,000 chemicals that are being added to our foods. The disturbing fact here is that most of them are not required to be listed on the label. Sadly,

The number of chemicals being used in our foods, toiletries and healthcare products alike is growing rapidly each year. It is, therefore, becoming increasingly difficult, if not impossible, to avoid toxic exposure. In a report published in 2005, the Environmental Working Group found an average of 200 industrial chemicals and pollutants in umbilical cord blood from 10 babies born in August and September of 2004 in U.S. hospitals[26]. It is a frightening and sickening fact that we are not only more toxic than those before us, we are even more toxic before we are born into this world.

The best way to keep your body in a toxic-free state is to avoid toxic exposure. Although there are certain exposures that will prove to be difficult to avoid, we will concern ourselves in this work with the factors that we can control. With that said, let's start with the largest organ in the body, your skin.

The skin is a very unique and complex organ. It is also one of the more difficult to maintain due to its increase in the exposure it receives from the environment, the array of beauty products we religiously apply to our skin, as well as the fact that it is the last area of the body to receive nourishment. You see, the body nourishes itself from the inside out. I am somewhat famous for repeatedly having said the following, "if your skin is in rough shape, I would hate to see what the rest of you looks like!" Of course, this is a generalized pun of sorts, but it is the basis of something that resides in truth.

---

[26] "Lead, mercury and cadmium in umbilical cord blood ... - NCBI." 12 Sep. 2013, https://www.ncbi.nlm.nih.gov/pmc/articles/PMC3848449/. Accessed 12 March. 2018.

In life, we are not always afforded as many choices as we think we are entitled to. As an individual, most do not have much control over the economy, the price of gas or the rising cost of insurance. The one thing that we have complete and utter control over, however, is what we choose to put into our mouth and apply to the surface of our skin. This choice starts with awareness, then leads to education and ultimately manifesting as a choice. Do not blindly throw foods into your cart without educating yourself and taking the time to research the foods you are feeding to yourself and to your family. There are free apps on the market today that can literally help you make point-of-sale decisions. As I write this I cannot help but wonder what the outcome has been given the fact that the majority of us have a world of information at our fingertips? I am not going to get in this in this particular work, however, this topic could be interesting for those of you searching for a school or work research project. If you do, I would love to learn of your findings!

In Ayurveda, they classify foods as we would classify medicines in the West. According to Ayurveda, medicines and foods are one in the same. We wouldn't, or shall I say most of us wouldn't shovel foreign pills into our mouths without first knowing what they are and what effect they'll have on our bodies and minds. Why then would you do the same with your foods? Most of the foods you consume regularly contain just as many chemicals as do the medications some of us are prescribed. It is a sad fact to face, but we are no longer consuming food, but rather chemically enhanced substances made to mimic, resemble and taste like food. The chemicals in our foods are causing inflammatory conditions, digestive disturbances and imbalances, skin issues and issues with our cognitive functions. Exhausting are the choices, the case studies, and the literature... this I know! I will teach you to understand the methods for playing it safe and eat foods grown naturally in nature. Locally grown produce is always the safest and best choice. Get out into your community, meet and talk to your local farmers!

There are many naturally occurring compounds that we can utilize in order to safely and effectively detoxify your body and mind. One of my favorites, though I would never recommend consuming it right before or during a date, are chia seeds. These little gelatinous scrubbers are one of the best and wholesome detoxifiers you can consume. They are abundant, inexpensive and are a very versatile food. Another is cilantro. Cilantro is an excellent detoxifier of mercury. It binds to the mercury atom and carries it safely out of your system. Cilantro is cooling in its nature and in moderation is good for all three of the *doshas*. You can incorporate cilantro into your salads, salsas, smoothies and raw juices. We will cover more natural detoxifiers and their qualities and uses later on, but for now, let's move on with this quote in mind: "If it is produced in a plant, avoid it. If it comes from a plant, consume it."

To Inflame or not to Inflame?

It has recently come out that one of the keys to Christie Brinkely and Tom Brady seemingly being timeless, is the fact that their diets are centered around foods that have inherent anti-inflammatory properties. Now, I am sure that most of my readers are not equipped with their vast resources, however, not having millions of dollars is surely not an excuse for consuming an improper diet. Do not buy into this fallacy!

Inflammation is a concern of epidemic proportions. Before we get into why it's bad and what you can do to thwart it, I think you need to first understand inflammation. When sensing danger your immune system, which primarily resides in the gut (we will get into and link this importance later), activates proteins that offer cell protection. Inflammation is a physiological response to something that the body views as being a threat. This, of course, can be viruses, bacteria, infections and toxic chemicals. Inflammation, though bad in its effect, is a protective mechanism of the body. Since it is a natural defense mechanism of the body, inflammation cannot fully be avoided, but it can be controlled. "In a healthy situation, inflammation serves as a good friend to our body," says Mansour Mohamadzadeh, PhD, director of the Center for Inflammation and Mucosal Immunology at the University of Florida." "But if immune cells start to overreact, that inflammation can be totally directed against us[27].

Some consider inflammation one of the primary factors in the disease process, and though I feel there are more underlying intricacies at play here, they are not far from the truth. More recently it has become a mystery symptom that is often times overlooked. Inflammatory consideration can be linked to a slew of emotional and physiological imbalance - ranging from skin conditions to

---

[27] "What Is Inflammation? 13 Ways it Affects Your Health | Health ...." 4 Mar. 2015, https://www.health.com/mind-body/13-ways-inflammation-can-affect-your-health. Accessed 6 April. 2018.

cancer. Not surprisingly, recent studies are popping up everywhere linking inflammation to even aspects of depression and other mental maladies. Inflammation, as most who suffer from it, know that it is a causative factor in fibromyalgia and other autoimmune diseases.

The Ayurvedic approach toward treating inflammation differs slightly from its counterpart here in the U.S. Inflammation is looked upon in Ayurveda as a result, not the cause. If you are experiencing any imbalances due to inflammatory conditions, the first thing you must do is to ask yourself what is causing the inflammation. Something you are consuming, doing, or even thinking is triggering an inflammatory response. Your emotional state and even your exercise routine could be potential triggers that we will examine in Part Two of this book. In simpler terms, everything you do, everything you consume and think is either inflammatory or anti-inflammatory. From this point forward, let's start looking upon inflammation as the signal or a sign that something you're doing or not doing is not fully agreeing with your body or mind. From there, we can use a systematic approach to eliminate the trigger(s). Here are a few more common triggers that you can start examining on your own:

1. **Stress** - Understanding your stress levels and what is causing you stress is a very important action you can take starting right now. Are you currently involved in toxic relationships that are causing you undue stress? For me it is watching any of my sports' teams lose or even perform poorly. This stress is certainly coming from

unwarranted means - means that I solely have the power to control. Knowing what causes you the most stress and implementing ways to avoid or lessen the stressors is one of the first steps you can take in eliminating inflammation.

2. **Reduce Inflammatory Foods** - After you reduce the stressors in your life, now it is time to eliminate food that is causing inflammatory conditions. Sugary foods are a good place to start. Not only do you need to look at white sugar, but more importantly you need to look at how much high fructose corn syrup you're consuming. I am willing to bet it's a leading contributor. It is the stuff is found in almost everything today. A high-fructose diet may induce inflammation as fructose accelerates renal disease in rats in association with an increase in monocyte-macrophage infiltration[28]. Most meats and foods that have been overprocessed will often produce an inflammatory response. Knowing which foods are inflammatory and which are anti-inflammatory may not help you throw a football as well as Tom Brady, but knowing this can certainly help you maintain a similar level of health and longevity.

There are, of course, more triggers for inflammation, but the above are two of the more common ones that you can start working to eliminate now. If there are any others, we can look at eliminating those in the custom version of this

---

[28] Gersch MS, Mu W, Cirillo P, Reungjui S, Zhang L, Roncal C, Sautin YY, Johnson RJ, Nakagawa T: Fructose, but not dextrose, accelerates the progression of chronic kidney disease. Am J Physiol Renal Physiol 293: F1256–F1261, 2007 [PubMed]

work. Just as there are foods that cause inflammation, there are also certain foods and herbs that are great at reducing inflammation. Here is a brief list of some of the best anti-inflammatory herbs used in Ayurveda:

- **Turmeric** - Is a staple in Ayurvedic medicine and cuisine alike. Turmeric is one of the most powerful anti-inflammatories known to man, as well as being effective in the treatment of over 500 maladies and imbalances. The active ingredient is called curcumin, or *curcuma longa*.
- **Ashwagandha** - In Ayurveda, ashwagandha is used and prescribed often. It's a common *rasayana* (blood purification) herb that is used for many health conditions. Clinical studies have shown it to relieve the pain of rheumatoid arthritis. Its naturally occurring steroidal content is even higher than that of hydrocortisone.
- **Guggul** - Guggul, for those of you unfamiliar with it, is made from the extract of a tree sap native to India. It's recommendations for arthritic conditions and arteriosclerosis and dates back in Ayurvedic literature to approximately 600 b.c[29]. It is most commonly found in capsule form.
- **Ginger** - Ginger, in addition to turmeric, is also an excellent herb for treating inflammatory disorders. Ginger, of course, is also an excellent digestive aid. Hence, why grandma used to always give you ginger ale for an upset stomach. In fact, a University of Miami study concluded that ginger extract could one day be a substitute to nonsteroidal.

---

[29] "Guggul Health Benefits - Ayurvedic Herbs | Banyan Botanicals." https://www.banyanbotanicals.com/info/plants/ayurvedic-herbs/guggulu/. Accessed 7 April. 2018.

anti-inflammatory drugs (NSAIDs). The study compared the effects of a highly concentrated ginger extract to placebo in 247 patients with osteoarthritis of the knee. The ginger reduced pain and stiffness in knee joints by 40 percent over the placebo[30].

- **Boswellia Serrata** - Boswellia is also known as Indian frankincense. It is an herbal extract taken from the *Boswellia serrata* tree. The resin from this tree, like guggul has been used for centuries in India, as well as in Asia and Africa. It is known for its anti-inflammatory properties and for treating numerous other health conditions like gum-related imbalances. It can be used in resin, pill or in cream form.

A Lemon or a Cupcake?

The above may seem like an obvious answer, but what would you say if I completed the title above by adding: "a lemon or a cupcake, which is more acidic?" The answer, surprising to most, is a cupcake. Like inflammation, everything you consume is either alkaline or acidic (note, some foods are neutral). Ironically, most foods that possess a high acidity level, are also the same foods that cause an increase of inflammation in the body. The Standard American Diet, in general, is loaded with foods which are far more acidic, creating an imbalance in the pH levels of your body. Current research has indicated that over 90% of the population here in the United States is far too acidic. The issue, however, lies at the duration in how long our bodies are living in a predominantly acidic state. Symptoms more commonly associated

---

[30] "Health Benefits of Ginger for Arthritis - Arthritis Foundation Blog." 22 Jan. 2016, http://blog.arthritis.org/living-with-arthritis/health-benefits-of-ginger/. Accessed 7 April. 2018.

with being too acidic are constantly feeling tired or exhausted and losing the luster of your hair and skin. Even being mentally exhausted can also be a strong indicator that your body is too acidic. Prolonged bad breath (halitosis), back pain, arthritic conditions and osteoporosis are just a few other manifestations one might experience when their diet is too acidic in nature. Most of these symptoms are also conditions in which inflammation is also a factor. The two often go hand-in-hand.

You always want to keep your body slightly more alkaline than acidic; 7.45 potential hydrogen is a general and healthy range. Under healthy conditions, the body will be slightly more alkaline. The stomach is the most acidic area of the body with a normal pH level of 3.5 or even slightly below so it can breakdown foods[31]. Processed and low quality foods keep us residing in an acidic state, thus allowing a host of different diseases to thrive - one being many forms of cancer. Sugary foods, as well as animal proteins and fats, yield an increase in the body's acidic levels. Soda is by far one of the most acidic things we regularly consume. Most sodas register around 2.3 on the pH scale (pH = potential hydrogen). The scary thing here, however, is that it takes 20 parts alkalinity to neutralize 1 part acidity. This means to neutralize a glass of cola with a pH of 2.5 you would need to consume 32 glasses of alkaline water with a pH of 10. Most tap waters come in around 6.0 on the pH scale. As an example, the average American consumes around 3 glasses of cola a day. This person would then need to consume around 96 glasses of alkaline water to return their body to a safe pH level. Not only would this, in and of itself, be

---

[31] "Gastric acid - Wikipedia." https://en.wikipedia.org/wiki/Gastric_acid. Accessed 7 April. 2018.

unhealthy (yes, you can consume too much water, especially for the *kapha dosha* type), but alkaline water is a bit pricey as well. The result, most won't do it - leaving themselves in a very acidic state and more susceptible to various diseases. So, you are probably wondering how can you easily return the body's pH level to the appropriate range of around 7.45? A good rule is what I call the 80/20: 80% of your foods should be alkaline, which would allow you to safely have 20% of your diet be more acidic in nature.

Foods which are alkaline are easy to decipher; pretty much everything green - especially leafy greens offer greater alkalinity. Here is a rule I used to teach in our Juice Jive classes; if it is the leaf, stem or flower it is most likely alkaline. If it is the root or animal flesh, it is acidic. Chlorella and spirulina (two forms of algae) are two of the most alkaline foods that you can consume. Most higher quality forms of these two nutrient powerhouses come in close to 11 on the pH scale. Wheatgrass is another high nutrient and very alkaline food you can consume. I recommend a 2 ounce shot of wheatgrass a day. If you are new to wheatgrass, start by consuming a shot a few times a week. Then increase your consumption to the 2 ounces a day. For your enjoyment and health, here is a very high alkaline smoothie recipe you can consume regularly to help counteract high levels of acidity:

- 8 ounces of alkaline water
- 1 serving spirulina or chlorella
- 1 green apple
- 1 thumb-sized knob of ginger, peeled

- Handful of baby spinach
- 1 tsp of turmeric
- ½ cup of pineapple

Not only is this remedy far healthier, it is also far less time consuming than sitting around and drinking 100 glasses of water every time you consume a few cups of coffee or a can of soda - talk about running to the restroom!

The Three Pillars of Health

"The three supports of life are....
Ahara – food, Nidra – sleep, and Brahmacharya – moderation of sexual intercourse

- Charaka sutra sthana, Chapter 11, verse 35

त्रय उपस्तम्भा इति– आहारः, स्वप्नो, ब्रह्मचर्यमिति;
एभिस्त्रिभिर्युक्तियुक्तैरुपस्तब्धमुपस्तम्भैः शरीरं
बलवर्णोपचयोपचितमनुवर्ततेयावदायुःसंस्कारात् संस्कारमहितमनुपसेवमानस्य , य
इहैवोपदेक्ष्यते॥३५॥

Triya Upstambha iti- Aaharah, swapno, brahmacharya miti, aibhistribhiryuktiyuktairupstabdhamupastambhayai shariram balvarnopchayopachitamnuvartateyaavadayu sanskaraat samskaramhitanupsevamanasya ya ihaivopdekshyate

Sleep, according to the Ayurvedic Scriptures is considered as one of the "Three Pillars" of health; nutrition and a balanced sexual drive being the other two. By being a basic instinct of life, an individual's pattern of sleep is determined by several unique criteria; their specific *doshic* makeup being the foundation of those particulars. Hemingway was quoted saying that when he is not sleeping his life has a tendency to fall apart. If you can recall, any disturbance of the *doshas* can begin to break down the equilibrium of the whole. Lack of sleep and or improper sleep has been proven in clinical studies to be a true causative factor of *doshic* aggravation. Studies here in the west have shown that sleep disorder is a serious issue for over 60% of Americans, who suffer respectively from nearly 70 different sleeping disorders[32]. The sad fact here, unfortunately, is that a sizable portion of those people are children. Growing up sleeping long undisturbed hours was merely a thing kids my age ritually performed. Has today's youth been robbed of that simple pleasure of being a kid?

A good night's sleep is nourishing and is a natural phenomena vital to all living things. Not only is proper sleep and the quality of sleep important, in Ayurveda, one's pattern of sleep is also an indicator of their current state of health (*vikriti*). Being used as a diagnostic tool, sleep can help lead the practitioner down the correct path towards uncovering the root cause(s) of the imbalance. Proper sleep is a vital function in relieving stress, and it is crucial in the formation of bodily tissues, such as muscular growth and development...just ask Arnold! Often being called the "great rejuvenator," your strength, cognitive function, endurance, immune function and overall level of happiness depends on it each and every night!

Speaking towards validating my earlier point regarding inflammation in Chapter 7, sleep is one of the best anti-inflammatories known to man - it has been since the conception of life. Creation, maintenance and elimination are the natural biological functions that are at play while we are asleep. Sleep is a time for regeneration and rejuvenation. During our deepest slumber, it is said that this is the time when our organs and tissues have a chance to detach from the grasp of our limited and biased egos, and they are afforded the chance to

---

[2] "Getting a good night's sleep - American Psychological."
https://www.apa.org/helpcenter/sleep-disorders. Accessed 8 April. 2018.

develop a greater connection to the Divine. It has even been recently proven in various sciences such as epigenetics, that our DNA communicates and receives information and instructions from, what Rupert Sheldrake coined as the morphogenic field. I will step out on a limb and say that when our bodies are not under the influence of our egoic, conscious minds while we are at sleep, the level of energetic communication between our bodies and the field is far greater and more efficient. By turning off the gatekeeper duties of the critical mind, our subconscious minds are more active and can communicate freely with this intelligent field that surrounds and encompasses all. This is the true source of wisdom and knowledge, not only for our minds, but for the trillions of cells of our bodies.

Causes of Poor Sleep

The root cause of your sleepless nights may seem to you as being as ambiguous as it is confusing. Do not fear! Do not lose another minutes sleep, for correcting this common imbalance is only a few chapters away. According to and keeping within the boundaries of the Ayurvedic model, all sleep-related issues are imbalances and physical manifestations of an aggravation of one's *dosha*. Remember, very seldom a time where the physical ailment or disorder is the root cause, it is most certainly always the effect. Let's take a deeper look into insomnia or as it is referred to in Ayurveda, *anidra*.

Understanding insomnia and what it means is often the first step towards overcoming it and allowing the body to return to its natural state. Insomnia lies so much deeper than not being able to sleep and extends into the depths of the nervous system where it can become weakened. There are several factors that contribute to insomnia. That's the bad news. The good news, however, is that most of the causes are lifestyle related, or as I simply call them, choices. Life is a never-ending swing of the pendulum and no longer will you feel compelled to make improper choices. As an example, abusing alcohol and drugs are often times at the helm of your sleepless nights. Anxiety and stressors are, of course, common everyday culprits. Like the choices you have regarding your diet, you are in control and are given the same birthright to choose something different regarding the factors causing your sleepless nights. By choosing something different the outcome will manifest as something different. This is law, and even our sleep cannot escape the law of cause and effect. You can start right now by identifying the cause of your sleepless nights. Here is a list of the more common causes, and though this is not nearly a complete list, it will help guide us towards uncovering the root cause of your insomnia, thus allowing you to finally experience a good night's rest.

- Too much caffeine, especially before bed
- Drugs & alcohol
- Stresses, such as work, family, financial and health related
- Overworked
- Trauma
- Ill health
- Emotional disorders, such as depression and anxiety
- Neurological disorders, such as Parkinson's & Alzheimer's

The Sub-doshas & Insomnia

Insomnia is classified into two categories; primary and secondary. The list above includes examples of both classifications of insomnia. In Ayurveda, insomnia is a disturbance of *tarpak kapha, sadhak pitta,* or *prana vayu (vata)*. The diagnostic functionality of Ayurveda is awesomely simplistic in its nature. We will delve further into the diagnostics of Ayurveda in a later chapter, but for now let's move on and look more closely at the insomnia and its relationship to the *tridoshas*.

It has been proven through Western modalities and countless case studies that deep sleep, often referred to as "R.E.M" allows for the body and mind to fully regenerate. This very closely relates to Ayurvedic model; only during the deeper levels of sleep can *ojas* be fully fabricated. Only when this is achieved can one experience a true state of health. *Ojas,* as you already know, is the conductor or the master coordinator between the mind, body and one's inner-self. It is the maintaining life force inherent within the body and mind, and when we are unable to achieve the proper state of sleep production of *ojas* is hampered, thus causing a multitude of physical and mental manifestations.

Prana Vayu

Prana vayu, a *subdosha* of *vata dosha,* regulates the nervous system and is a sensitive component of its proper functioning. When you are experiencing an increase of anxiety or stress, this surely creates an imbalance within *prana vayu*, thus manifesting as sleeplessness or insomnia. The sleeping pattern of a person who is predominantly of this *dosha* or is experiencing a disruption of this *dosha*, is easy to spot. A light sleep that is often erratic and easily disturbed are strong indicators. Needing prolonged sleep is a very important aspect of this person's daily and nightly routine that will need to be developed over time, and a person of this nature will benefit from longer sleep times than that of the other *doshas*. Due to an excess of protruding bones, a softer sleeping surface is welcomed, as well as a dark and very quiet environment.

Sleep Requirement: 6 to 7 hours per night

Sadhak Pitta

Located within the heart *sadhaka pitta* is an auxiliary of the *pitta dosha*[33]. It is known to control our deepest desires and deepest impulses. Overworking and demanding behaviors are symptoms often exhibited by someone who is suffering from an imbalance of *sadhka pitta*, thus ultimately causing insomnia. By sleeping more easily and deeper than the *vata dosha*, the *pitta dosha* will require cooler sleeping environments. Take it from a true *pitta*, the hot and muggy nights of the summer months are our foe and do lend to a lower quality of sleep. While experiencing an increased level of the fire element, as well as being overly engaged in a task that has aroused their inner creativity, sleep can and often times is limited. With that said, however, for shorter periods of time, foregone sleep is okay for this *dosha*. Fiery and active

---

[33] "Sadhaka Pitta – Location, Functions, Imbalance, Disorders ...." 19 Dec. 2018, https://easyayurveda.com/2018/12/19/sadhaka-pitta/. Accessed 8 April. 2018.

dreams are often accompanied with deeper states of sleep and reaching sufficient periods of R.E.M is crucial for the transformation and processing of psychological and mental issues that need to be resolved. If you're *pitta* in nature and feel more creative at night, then roll with it and allow this true aspect of your specific nature to shine brilliantly. You will notice an increased in the flow of creativity during these times. I am typing this for you at 2:38am.

Sleep Requirement: 7 to 8 hours per night

Tarpak Kapha

One of the main functions of this auxiliary *dosha* of *kapha* is to properly nourish the cells of the brain. When proper cell nourishment is not achieved brain fog is often experienced, thus causing a decrease in mental clarity and sharpness, as well as sleepless nights. When this *dosha* is out of balance insomnia is often a physical manifestation. The prolonged and heavy nature of the *kapha dosha* is an unmistakable trait. They love to sleep and will sleep as often as they can and will experiencing long, deep and uninterrupted sleeping patterns. Managing their periods and length of sleep becomes important, but not an easy accomplish task. Ironically, they have the greatest tendency to oversleep out of the three body-types, and as I mentioned before, they need to get up and get things moving! By experiencing calm and normal dreams, as well as preferring a softer and comfier surface, this is one area of health that is normally not a concern. If you feel you are *kapha dosha*, begin to imagine ways to lessen the amount of your sleep and how you can increase your activity levels. Of course, we will go over the specifics for you in the last part of this work.

Sleep Requirement: 7 to 8 hours per night

Treatment of Insomnia

As a first step, understanding the true root cause of insomnia is the only effective way to begin to uncover the root cause of this common imbalance. Once this has been properly established, and of course, knowing one's specific *dosha*, there are several very effective modalities that can be employed. Each course of treatment is based solely on which *subdosha* has been disturbed, and it is here where the precise treatment will be used to bring one's *doshic* state into balance. Here are generalized examples for each of the three auxiliary *doshas*:

Prana Vayu - Administering *ashwagandha*, an herb which is an adaptogen, will help decrease increased cortisol levels when there is an elevation of the *vata dosha*.

Sadhak Pitta - Controlling the elevation of the fire element becomes critical when dealing with a vitiation of the *pitta dosha*. Cooling foods, tulsi tea, as well as a coconut oil self-massage (*abhyanga*).

Tarpak Kapha - *Abhyanga* can also be employed for a disturbance of this *dosha*, however, a heating oil such as mustard would need to be used. Detox treatments such as *Shirodhara*, an important step of *panchakarma* (the five actions) has been very effective in treating the vitiation of *tarpak kapha*.

Mental & Spiritual Functions of Sleep

To sum up the most important aspect of sleep in one single sentence would be to say that there are certain aspects that the body needs to achieve that it cannot otherwise achieve during the awakened state of consciousness. There are, of course, many benefits of proper sleep. Some are easily defined and studied, while there are others that fall under the black cloud of the ethereal and the esoteric. They are, nonetheless, important and need to be properly understood.

One aspect of sleep that is more difficult to explain, are dreams. Most dreams go unremembered or are viewed as having no actual significance in our lives, especially towards one's overall well-being. There are some who would strongly disagree with this consensus, and in certain cultures a God of Sleep is religiously worshiped. The altered state of consciousness that is achieved during sleep, which is similar in its nature to certain aspects of hypnotic trance, has been revered for many generations in indigenous cultures for allowing one great access to Divine insight[34]. After all, aren't dreams the

---

[34] "Brain Oscillations, Hypnosis, and Hypnotizability - NCBI." 13 Jan. 2015, https://www.ncbi.nlm.nih.gov/pmc/articles/PMC4361031/. Accessed 9 April. 2018.

language of the soul? In the ancient Yogic traditions, a sound and deep sleep shares many common aspects with that of *Samadhi*, which is a highly revered state of mind that is thought to be achieved only through deeper states of meditation, which is beyond the capacity of the conscious, rational mind.

Pillar Two: Sex Drive

By developing, understanding and incorporating each aspects of the Three Pillars of Health, one can experience true happiness and longevity. One aspect of these timeless and ancient traditions is the importance that it places upon an over-indulgence in any area of the Three Pillars. This next pillar for most, could just be a "touchy" subject. And to those who are already beginning to blush, this chapter is not about sex in the literal sense, though if it were I would perhaps sell far more copies.

Creating a sense of balance within the walls of these pillars is critical for residing within the boundaries of true health and wellness. By not recognizing both their importance and their delicate interplay, a myriad of issues can arise, from headaches to infertility. One underlying principle of Ayurveda is the fact that it places the importance and responsibility of the individual to oversee and participate in their own affairs and their overall well-being. Would you agree that the common consensus today is the polar opposite; I'll do what I want, when I want and how much of it I want, regardless of the result. When the situation gets out of control and sickness ensues, a pill or surgery are the default choices. Does that sound about right? What is your feeling towards your responsibilities towards your overall health? Once you come to know and understand the natural rhythms of the bio-forces of life, you can then take that most important first step towards becoming the master of your domain, and no longer will you fall victim to the effect or the consequence of your past choices or mistakes.

By managing the pendulum swings between wholesome and unwholesome, you can begin to apply it to every aspect of your daily life. Everything in life is a choice and these choices carry with them the law of cause and effect; bringing forth immediate and long term manifestations based solely upon the mental creation of each thought. I am here to tell you that your sex life is no different and must be handled in the same manner as your dietary, exercise and sleep routines.

The Ayurvedic philosophy is built upon the premise that the human body is constructed from seven tissues (*dhatus*); the first being plasma, which creates the sexual fluids, or as it is referred to in Ayurveda, *shukra dhatu*. The process to go from food-stuff to plasma to the seventh *dhatu* takes approximately one month. Being created from aspects of the *rasa dhatu*, it is easy to see how our dietary choices directly affect our sexual drive and production, as well as performance. In addition, *apana vayu*, or as I have often called it the "5 winds," is directly responsible for the regulation of the menstruation cycle, reproduction and even the orgasm. If the movement of *vayu* is fluid and strong, sexual desires and production will manifest in a like manner.

In recent years there has been an increase in articles stating the importance and benefits of experiencing an orgasm has on the body. Things that make you go, Hmmm, for sure, but is there scientific proof supporting their claims? And what is the Ayurvedic point of view regarding orgasms? Does having an orgasm in fact release stress? Can it boost immunity, as well as increase the production of oxytocin? The short answer is yes, but in the eyes of the Yogi, it may not be that easy or that black and white.

One main factor that you need to consider regarding the effect an orgasm has on your body relates to the timeless and relentless law of cause and effect. You see, experiencing an orgasm, especially often, increases the air element in the body, thus creating an excess and ultimately causing a vitiation of *vata dosha*. Excessive orgasms can be depleting to the body and must be managed like every other aspect of our lives. In more scientific terms, the release of sexual fluids is an actual process of depletion; a process that takes the human body a month to make. Are you starting to understand the importance of managing a state of balance? This, in turn, limits and decreases the production of *ojas*. Every effect has a cause and every cause has a similar effect. There is no avoiding this and ignorance towards it only exasperates the conditions.

Just as consuming meals at certain times of the day is recommended, having sex at certain times of day is just as important. The best time of day to engage in sexual activity is during the day. Now, this of course, is not a prescription to find a quiet place at the office and have a quickie with a coworker. The morning time right after sunrise is also recommended, but just make sure you do "it" by 10 a.m. And sadly for you night owls, having sex or even masturbation is not advised at night. Perhaps a good book will help...

I know, you're probably wondering at this point how often is enough and is there such a thing as "too much sex"? Well, I am here to tell you more is not necessarily better. There are many factors to consider regarding sexual frequency as well as sexual intensity. From the time of day, as I just mentioned, to seasonality, and of course, the overall health of the individual and the current state of their *doschic* make-up. Someone in a good state of health with strong *ojas* and engaging in sex during the early spring and winter months can welcome sexual encounters 3-5 times a week. Preferably, of course, with the same sexual partner. When summer and autumn dawns our days, you horny birds will need to drop that to approximately 1-2 times a week. During the times of year where it is recommended to engage in greater sexual frequency, you can incorporate food that will help in the production of *shukra dhatu* as well as build *ojas*, such as coconut milk and juice, as well as ghee. As a tip, and ironically it is also recommended in Ayurveda, begin each encounter with the practice of massage and gently applying oils before sex. Trust me, both your body and partner will thank you!

According to the underlying philosophies of Ayurveda, the main goal of life is sovereignty over the Three Pillars of Health, which when understood correctly, intertwines the fabric of your overall level of well-being and happiness. Most have heard the term Kama Sutra which in Vedic traditions is both romantic and sexual love, as well as any related pleasures, was ironically penned in its entirety by a lifelong celibate monk[35]. I guess no longer am I able to knock my high school hockey coach for not being able to skate.

The oftentimes hidden premise lying beneath the sexual allure of the *Kama Sutra* is that of the unique relationship between the *Kama Sutra, the Dharma and the Arthra*. They need to be separately understood, yet the delicate balance between them needs attention and certainty. With any aspect of our lives, when striving for fulfillment in one area, we are to never neglect fulfillment in the others. Our sexuality as humans and its erotic nature is something that humans need to integrate into their lives and properly fulfill. By understanding the subtler aspects of the *Kama Sutra, the Dharma and the Arthra*, we can begin to specifically balance each aspect into our lives, never neglecting one for the singular benefit of another. As we continue to build a deeper understanding while proceeding into the last half of this work, we will take an individual look at learning how to balance these three keys aspects of living as well as deepening our understanding.

---

[35] "Kama Sutra - Mindvalley Blog." 9 Oct. 2018, https://blog.mindvalley.com/kama-sutra/. Accessed 11 April. 2018.

Personalize Your Life with Ayurveda

By understanding your true nature and the vital aspects that make up your unique constitution, even your personal relationships will improve. Ayurveda suggests a spouse of a different constitution. By choosing a spouse of a predominantly different *dosha*, you are in fact creating a sense of balance within your life. This can help prevent your children from being too extreme in any one *dosha*. Two parents with a *kapha dosha* dominance will produce a child who is doubly *kapha*, for example. You will, of course, want to always follow your heart when choosing a lifelong partner, but there are simple and easy to follow criteria that can help increase the odds of longevity and your overall happiness. With that said, below is a chart for quick reference in helping you understand the delicate intricacies that exist when choosing a life partner. Perhaps Paula Abdul was right, opposites do attract, and they should. Or do they...?

Balancing Kapha	**Balancing Pitta**	**Balancing Vata**
Marry *Vata* or *Pitta*	Marry *Kapha* or *Vata*	Marry *Kapha* or *Pitta*
Active Family life	Soothing Conversations	Slow and Steady
Stimulating Conversations	Little to no Confrontation	Less Thinking, More Acting
Encourage Talking	Relaxing Massages	Careful Managing Money

Go out and Get Interested	Take "Cool off" Breaks	Commitment
Encourage Sexual Interest	Slow Down and Cool off to Take Time and Care for Sex	Consistent and Supportive Behavior Caution w/ Sexual Experimentation

The definition of fulfillment within the scope of Ayurveda is quite clear and concise; a satisfying sexual union embraces health and vitality upon you and your partner. It is essential that both partners are satisfied. Engaging in or routinely practicing deviant or unsatisfying sexual behaviors can and does have an adverse effect on both the mental and physical planes of health. It aggravates the *doshas* and reduces immunity function, just to name a few. Oh, and don't forget to urinate after sex!

The last Pillar of Health under the realm and science of Ayurveda is nutrition. Since nutrition was one of my main motivators for writing this book, as well as given the fact that I have and will sprinkle the various aspects of nutrition throughout this work, I am not going to get into this pillar specifically in this section. With that said, let's move on...

Ayurveda and the Mind

> *"Thinking is an object for the mind (it can be observed).*
> *Thus the wrong use of the mind creates abnormal mental conditions.*
> *The right use of the mind creates mental stability."*
>
> - Charaka Sutrasthana, Chapter 8, verse 16

विचार मन के लिए एक वस्तु है (इसका अवलोकन किया जा सकता है)। इस प्रकार मन का गलत उपयोग असामान्य मानसिक स्थिति पैदा करता है। मन का सही उपयोग मानसिक स्थिरता बनाता है

> **vichaar man ke lie ek vastu hai,**
> **(isaka avalokan kiya ja sakata hai).**
> **is prakaar man ka galat upayog asaamaany**
> **maanasik sthiti paida karata hai.**
> **man ka sahee upayog maanasik sthirata banaata hai**

Maintaining the delicate dance between mind, body and soul is not only the ultimate goal in Ayurveda, when achieved it is also considered to be complete health. Do all diseases have as their root cause an imbalance of the mind? Do the ancient traditions of Ayurveda coincide with the current viewpoint of quantum energy and its relationship to the mind and body? It has been said that everything we witness in the outer world started as a thought. If this is true, are the sick and dying a mere reflection of this attitude?

Ayurveda is the science of life and thus, has its own identity when compared to other modern systems of healthcare. By dealing with the whole being from the moment of conception until the moment of death, this unique system of health emphasizes its treatment modalities into three unique, but yet, integrated parts; psychotherapy (*Sattvavajaya Chikitsa*), divine medicine (*Daivyapashray chikitsa*) and tactical therapy (*Yuktivyapashray chikitsa*). By being the functional element of the soul (*Atman*), the mind in Ayurveda predates the vedic period. Does this perhaps tell us something of the importance in which our minds play in our overall level of our health and longevity?

The existence of psychotherapy can be found in most every system of healthcare in the world today, even though Ayurveda's take is quite different from the days of Freud. Caraka states, as in the quote above, that "thinking is an object," and therefore we cannot be our thoughts for they can be observed. This is such a powerful point and urges us to create a state of dissociation when looking upon our thoughts, feelings and emotions. They are not us - they belong to us. If in fact this is true, and we have domain over our possessions, doesn't it stand to reason that we can move or remove, gather and disperse them whenever we choose? Just by adjusting my mind to understand the true nature of this point sends a wave of relief throughout my body. We are not our psychology, but rather it belongs to us. No longer do we need to be a slave to our thoughts, feelings and emotions; for now we can move forward being their master.

When dealing with the mind, the systematic approach of Ayurveda builds upon that of the previous chapters on the 5 elements, the biological humors (*doshas*) and the *gunas*. Moving forward based upon this understanding will allow you to delve deeper into your own levels of awareness, thus helping to bridge the gap between your inner and outer worlds - inner and outer minds. When dealing with matters of consciousness and that which is unseen, it can be difficult to digest. I'll be the first to admit that it takes more than merely reading the words to fully understand the true meaning. May I suggest meditation?

I need to take a moment here to elaborate further on a few terms which I will use throughout this chapter and beyond in order to limit the amount of miscommunication. When speaking of "consciousness" I am referring to the energetic aspects of the mind. This aspect is far more subtle than our modern understanding of the word and may take a few moments of quiet introspection to fully grasp. From here, consciousness can be divided into two parts; habituated and unhabituated. Habituated consciousness is our unique collections of all of our past memories, thoughts, experiences and beliefs. From this storehouse of data, our unconscious beliefs are embedded into the fabric of the mind, thus controlling over 90% of our daily behaviors and beliefs.

The habituated aspect of the mind in Ayurveda is referred to as *manas*. Stimulus from the external world is perceived via the five senses, from which this information is thus processed by *manas*. You can liken *manas* to the id or ego. Through *manas,* we can perceive and observe our thoughts, feelings and other subtler objects. These objects are then transmitted and processed by *buddhi*, which is the aspect that decides on the appropriate actions. This is similar to the relationship between the conscious and unconscious mind, however, Ayurveda is built upon a much more comprehensive foundation. It is of no surprise to understand why Caraka is quoted saying, "the wrong use of mind creates abnormal conditions, where the right use of mind creates mental stability[36]."

When looking at our unhabituated consciousness we step into far more universal and much subtler aspects of mind. The unhabituated consciousness is our true self without the limitations of our past experiences, biases and memories encompassing all levels of the mind. It is through the unhabituated aspects of mind where we are able to connect to the Divine. Being free from all the prejudices of our habituated consciousness will allow you to tap the reservoir of deeper learning, knowledge and of true wisdom.

Any minor disturbances within the mind can create a windfall of future complications, thus manifesting both mentally and physiologically. When looking at the three *gunas* of the mind, Ayurveda states disease can stem from a disturbance of any of the three *gunas;* named as balance (*satwa*), arrogance (*raja*) *and* indolence (*tama*). The three *gunas* being the reactive aspects of the mind, are sensitive to any vitiation, thereby cultivating a healthy mind will help you establish wellness within the body and within the mind. The three

---

[36] "Ayurvedic Psychology - Vaidya Atreya Smith."
http://www.atreya.com/ayurveda/Ayurvedic-Psychology.301.html. Accessed 7 May. 2018.

psychological *gunas* are often referred to as the clearness and darkness of the mind. You are aware of, or should be aware by now, that any accumulation of toxins within the three *doshas* is the root cause of all disease. The mind is no different, but instead of being physiological contaminants, they consist of emotional and other mental toxins. If left unattended, they will ultimately manifest as some sort of mental or physical malady.

If these mental toxins, or when looking upon them in a more direct manner, these negative emotions are not properly or fully processed, they begin to create minor disturbances in one or more of the *gunas*. Repressed emotions, any traumatic experience that is not allowed to be processed and released then becomes the root cause of all mental imbalances, which sadly, can and does manifest in the physical body. If these emotional toxins are left unresolved for long periods of time they can give rise to a slew of physical disorders such as anxiety, depression, neurosis and insomnia, just to name a few.

Operations of the Mind

The mind, after receiving stimulus from the external world via the five human senses, interprets the bits or packets of information. This is the inner workings of *manas*: to perceive, interpret and develop the information. In Sanskrit, this is termed as *samskara*. The habituated aspects of the mind, or as Frawley states in "Ayurveda and the Mind," the conditioned mind, acts as a catalyst between the bits of information coming in through the senses and the bits that are ultimately processed. The aspects of *manas* can be likened to the conscious mind in western modalities, and as in today's understanding this is where the weakness exists; the habituated mind or *manas* bases its selection upon our past experiences, beliefs and limited biasess. As stimuli is perceived through the senses, the habituated mind then begins a search of matching that data to the records of our past. As a result of this internalized process of selection, the stimuli is then deleted, generalized and often distorted to fit our understanding of the world around us. As an example, if I am a professional athlete, I will unknowingly bend the stimuli coming in through my senses to fit my engrained sports minded model of reality. If I am a sculptor, the same internalization will happen to sculpt reality to fit my artistic viewpoint. And so on and so on...

The brilliance of this interplay of minds fascinates me still to this day. When the information coming in through the five senses is beyond the selection processing capabilities of the habituated mind (*manas*), the unhabituated mind or the unconscious aspects of the mind kicks in to help out. If any of the information is not able to be processed by the habituated mind, the information is thus sent to the unconscious mind. It is here, at this level of mind where continued searches and processing continues. The balanced nature of the *buddhi* has the capacity to process many times the amount of information than the *manas* can handle. In addition, it has more of a direct access to the Universal Mind and often correlates the information at this level of truth and understanding. This is one of the exact reasons why the famous hypnotist, Milton H. Erikson, was so successful in treating the untreatable; his utilization approach to hypnosis which fostered many forms of confusion, puns, metaphors and stories was far too much for the conscious reasoning of his clients minds. This provided him a direct window into the unhabituated aspects of their minds. Did you ever experience a situation where you are sure you know something but for whatever reason you cannot put your finger on it? Several minutes later, and always out of the blue, the thing you were trying to remember pops into your mind? Most have, yes! The unconscious mind continues the search for the answer for up to 10-15 minutes after your conscious awareness has given up and switched focus. This area of the mind is what is considered as the unhabituated mind, and it was at this level of mind that allows hypnotherapy to be successful on many levels.

Psychotherapy, the Ayurvedic Take

The process of bringing the intellect, the fortitude and the memory of the person into a balanced state is the ultimate goal of Ayurveda's approach to mental wellness. There are two processes through which this transpires: (1) assurance to the patient of the return of lost objects or bits and packets of information. (2) the inducement of emotions of an opposite nature to those emotions currently being experienced by the patient[37]. These techniques that form the basis for psychotherapy within the Ayurvedic model closely matches that of both Gestalt Therapy and the utilization approach taken by Erikson. This modality is a practice, like hypnosis, that can be administered by oneself or by one's family, community or by a practitioner specializing in mediations of the mind within the realms of the unseen. Caraka speaks of "objective"

---

[37] "Ayurvedic concepts related to psychotherapy - NCBI." https://www.ncbi.nlm.nih.gov/pmc/articles/PMC3705701/. Accessed 7 May. 2018.

mind control involving the physician's interference, thus ultimately saying that in *sattvavajaya* a physician wins the mind of the patient[38]. It is interesting to know that *sattvavajaya* translates into "the conquest of mind".

By beginning to understand that the mind and body form an integral system, only then can you understand the importance of treating any disorders of a spiritual or mental nature first. In the Upanishads, it is said that the mind is sensitive in its nature; even diet will change or impact the psychology. That is the bad news, of course. The good news, however, is minor changes of an opposite nature can impact the mind positively. It is important to understand the pendulum swings easily in both directions. Dr. Marc Halpern describes the origination of all mental illness as a lack of clarity[39]. Lack of clarity, is perhaps a bit ambiguous, but it directly relates to the true nature of balance. We've discussed earlier in this chapter that emotions are viewed as being objects within the Ayurvedic model, so it stands to reason that when one is experiencing emotions of a negative nature they cause a lack of mental clarity, or the ability to view one's true self. Experiencing emotions like greed, fear, anger, hate and jealousy will begin to expose the oversensitive nature of the mind, and as I stated earlier, will begin to accumulate as toxins of the mind. If left ignored or unattended, they will manifest as a disease of the mind, body or both.

---

[38] Jean, M. - Ayurvedic Psychotherapy: Transposed Signs. Langford: Parodied Selves; [Google Scholar]

[39] Dr. Marc Halpern, *Principles of Ayurvedic Medicine: Tenth Edition* (September, 2010), p.190

Treatment of Psychological Disorders

Ayurveda endeavors to treat the energetic factors of disease and it surely doesn't stray from this timeless concept when looking to treat imbalances of the mind. Its beauty lies in this simplistic approach; a dull mind you make sharp. An overly sharp mind you counteract by employing that of dullness. The process of restoring the proper balance of the mind is to cultivate clarity in the mind, this we now know. Clarity of the mind is referred to as *sattva* in Ayurveda. A dull or lethargic mind will possess higher qualities of the *kapha dosha*, so revving up the mind with intellectual activities of an energetic and fiery nature will restore balance by introducing the opposite nature of the imbalance.

The first step is to determine which *guna* is most prominent, just as in assessing your dominant *dosha*. If your mind is *tamasic*, then you'll need to cultivate aspects of a *rajasic* nature to offer a counterbalance to reduce the mental stagnation. Spending time in nature, meditation, yoga and greatly reducing the amount of negative stimulus, like watching disturbing news, will create a *rajasic* nature of mind. Yes, to most this may seem like a difficult or even tedious task, but rest assured, nothing could be further from the truth. As an example, one of the most profound ways to foster a balanced mind and build *ojas* is to engage in a balancing routine. In Ayurveda the importance of cultivating a *doshic* specific routine is so important that there exists a system of cultivation called *dinacharya*. This, in a nutshell, is the premise of this entire work and will be the main focus moving forward. In circadian medicine, an emerging medicine that delves into the molecular and genetic underpinnings of circadian rhythms and looks at the impacts of disruption in our biological clocks in health and disease, shows how our bodies and minds revolve around a 24-hour cycle. Newer studies in this promising field have shown that misalignment in the circadian rhythms is linked to depression, bipolar and schizophrenia[40]. An erratic sleeping routine can be a cause of unbalanced circadian rhythms. Sleep as you now know is a critical aspect to one's daily routine that should be *doshic* specific and should be religiously performed.

Nutrition and the Mind

We've known for quite some time that the food we consume is broken down in the body as useful substances which nourish bone and tissue, as well as cellular reproduction. Unbeknownst to most, and this is where the Ayurvedic differs from the mainstream sciences of today, what we consume is also broken down into the energetic factors of *tamas, rajas and sattva*. When looking at diet, eating foods that are balancing to your *dosha* and your mental constitution is not only healthy for your body, but is also a must for your mind. According to Dr. Frawley, *rajasic* and *tamasic* foods create a disruption of the mind and can cause unrest and disease. Consuming a diet of a *sattvic* nature aids in the treatment of psychological and mental maladies due to the fact that they restore harmony and balance of the mind[41]. Foods that have

---

[40] "Links between Circadian Rhythms and ... - NCBI - NIH." 6 May. 2014, https://www.ncbi.nlm.nih.gov/pmc/articles/PMC4018537/. Accessed 7 Jan. 2020.

[41] David Frawley, *Ayurveda and the Mind: The Healing of Consciousness* (Lotus Press, 1997) p. 103

been overcooked, microwaved, reheated, frozen or processed or highly refined are void of the life essence called *Prana*, and therefore are *rajasic* in nature. Fresh foods, fruits, vegetables and organic whole grains are examples of *sattvic* foods. Meat and other animal products, onions, garlic and mushrooms are considered dark in nature or *tamasic*, and therefore should be greatly reduced or even eliminated for certain *doshic* types and at certain times of the year. Issues such as these will be specifically designed for you in your customized version of this work.

Looking at the importance of diet and its relationship to mental health is no longer a lost science. Western scientists of today are now on board with this crucial aspect of mental health. A 2014 review of the emerging field of nutritional psychiatry states, "research suggests that nutrition not only matters directly with regard to the conditions treated within various medical disciplines but also has the potential to influence mental outlook and mental disorders. We cannot ignore this, particularly as it is becoming increasingly clear that diminished mental outlook and elevated perceptions of stress are drivers of unhealthy eating habits"[42]. Does this not say the same thing stated by Caraka, but only in the language of our time today? Does not a "diminished mental outlook" suggest a lack of mental clarity?

---

[42] "Nutritional psychiatry research: an emerging discipline ... - NCBI." 24 Jul. 2014, https://www.ncbi.nlm.nih.gov/pmc/articles/PMC4131231/. Accessed 12 May. 2018.

Stimuli, food for the Mind

The foods we consume nourish our bodies, well, that is the goal. The external impressions we perceive also nourish. What you perceive either nourishes the energetic aspects of the mind or they create a disturbance. This is not the only similarity between the mind and the body. Just as the foods you consume need to be properly digested, assimilated and eliminated, so does the sensory input that's being received via your five senses. We are continually being exposed to chemicals via the olfactory sense, as well as fluorescent lights, loud music and background noises. All of this sensory input must be progressed and digested by our nervous system before it can be interpreted by the mind. Therefore, the goal of an Ayurvedic lifestyle, as well as the goal of your individual lifestyle should be that of consuming foods nourishing to the mind, body and soul. The senses can be used as a form of medicine when sensory impressions are consciously chosen or as poison when sensory impressions are driven by desires and addictions.

Now, with this said, I am a realist and live in the modern world here in the West that is dominated by our fast-paced and hectic daily lives, filled with mobile electronic devices and overpriced stimulants. Trying to ensure that 100% of all foods and external stimuli is nourishing and balancing is a very difficult task. Yes, trying to accomplish this in and of itself can be taxing and very stressful. I am a firm believer, however, that ensuring that the majority is nourishing and balancing to your mental and physiological makeup is not only achievable, but becomes a must. Here is a fact most of us overlook; it is much easier and far less expensive to keep ourselves in a state of balanced equilibrium than it is to return oneself back from a state of disease. Ask anyone suffering from cancer or type 1 diabetes, especially those without the fortune of having applicable healthcare.

Below is a chart based upon the work of Dr. Frawley. The simplistic nature of these lifestyle recommendations should be as rewarding as they're easily incorporated. Again, these recommendations are a general guide. For your specific and unique psycho-physiological makeup, a more precise application may be needed.

	Vata	Pitta	Kapha
Sound	Calming music: classical, chanting or peaceful silence	Cooling and soft music: flute, water sounds	Stimulating music, strong energizing sounds
Touch	Gentle warming touch or massage using warm oils like sesame or almond	Cooling, soft and moderate touch with cooling oils like coconut or sunflower	Strong, deep body massage with dry powders and stimulating oils like mustard
Sight	Bright, calming colors like gold, orange, blue, green and white	Cool colors like white, blue and green	Bright, stimulating colors like yellow, orange, gold and red
Taste	Rich and nourishing food abounding in sweet, salty and sour tastes, with moderate use of spices	Food that is neither too heavy nor too light, abounding in sweet, bitter and astringent tastes, with cooling spices like coriander, turmeric and fennel	Light diet emphasizing pungent, bitter and astringent tastes with liberal use of spices, occasional fasting

	Vata	Pitta	Kapha
Smell	Sweet, warm, calming and clearing fragrances like jasmine, rose, sandalwood, eucalyptus	Cool and sweet fragrances like rose, sandalwood, vetivert, champak, gardenia and jasmine	Light, warm, stimulating and penetrating fragrances like musk, cedar, myrrh, camphor and eucalyptus

Yoga and the Mind

It has been known for many generations that physical exercise is a great release of emotional stress. It can serve as an emotional catalyst to help us process any excess sentiment. This is largely due to the fact that the mind and body are in constant connection. How you feel physically determines how your feel mentally. How you feel mentally determines how you feel physically. It's a never-ending cycle of influence and there is no human being that can escape this law of nature. So, how do you easily balance this mental, physical and emotional interplay? One easy way is the incorporation of yoga. The art and science of yoga is a timeless tradition of Ayurveda. According to Halpren, "Yoga is defined as calming the disturbances of the *chitta*, which are called *chitta vritti*, and in this regard, classical yoga is a psychology. Defined as a means of alleviating, mental psychological and emotional suffering[43]. Classical yoga, or as it is referred, *ashtanga*, involves a foundation of the 8 limbs:

---

[43] Frawley, David, and Marc Halpern. *Ayurvedic Psychology: Anxiety and Depression*. Rec. 18 Nov. 2006. California College of Ayurveda, 2006. CD.

1. **Yama** – Rules of Social Conduct
2. **Niyama** – Rules of Personal Behavior
3. **Asana** – Physical Postures: Right Orientation of the Physical Body
4. **Pranayama** – Breath Control: Right Use of the Vital Force
5. **Pratyahara** – Control of the Mind and Senses
6. **Dharana** – Concentration: Control of Attention
7. **Dhyana** – Meditation: Right Reflection
8. **Samadhi** – Absorption: Right Union

Frawley states that mental misalignment and disruption is merely a misuse of the subtler forms of mental energies. Happiness and unhappiness are the end results of the delicate balance and interplay of the energetic factors of the body and the mind. They affect the whole, hence why Ayurveda is considered a holistic form of medicine and healthcare. Your *doshic* makeup as well as your psyche pervade your entire being, therefore, when looking at health and disease as a whole you have to consider all encompassing aspects of your whole. The art of yoga is based upon an inner integration of reestablishing the union between the Trinity, not to mention its many physical benefits like spine and joint realignment. In an article published by The American Psychological Association, they stated that "There is a growing body of research documenting yoga's psychological benefits." According to Dr. Sat Bir Khalsa, neuroscientist, professor of medicine at Harvard Medical School at Brigham and Women's Hospital in Boston, and a leading researcher in the field, "Yoga targets unmanaged stress, a main component of chronic disorders such as anxiety, depression, obesity, diabetes and insomnia. It does this by reducing the stress response, which includes the activity of the sympathetic nervous system and the levels of the stress hormone cortisol. The practice enhances resilience and improves mind-body awareness, which can help people adjust their behaviors based on the feelings they're experiencing in their bodies"[44].

Again, the main concept here that must be fully understood is that man is not a machine and as such can't be operated equally with a uniform law. Change one aspect of the mind and body and affect the whole. This is law and it is inescapable. A verse from the *Yoga Sutra*, *Yogas Vritti Nirodhana*, describes yoga as a settled state of mind[45]. This is comparable to the Ayurvedic treatise, which states that one who remains united with the Self is considered a healthy person. Since the ultimate goal is identical, does it make sense to utilize the positive mental, physiological and emotional benefits of yoga? Mantras are sacred sounds that are known to impact our vibration, frequency, and energy at a cellular level and may offer a vital role in healing the body, mind and spirit. Mantras are often chanted in Sanskrit, and are designed to be *dosha* specific. We will look more closely at your unique situation in your customized version to see if and what form of yoga and mantras will be best suited for you to incorporate into your daily routine.

---

[44] Novotney, Amy. "Yoga as a Practice Tool." *Monitor on Psychology* 40, no. 10 (November 2009): 38. doi:10.1037/e598452009-018. http://www.apa.org/monitor/2009/11/yoga.aspx

[45] "Intro to Yoga Philosophy: Sutra School 1.2 - Yoga Journal." 28 Aug. 2007, https://www.yogajournal.com/yoga-101/intro-to-yoga-philosophy-sutra-school-1-2. Accessed 12 May. 2018.

Herbs and the Mind

I am sure you've heard countless times from your parents or guardians to "eat all your veggies." I am definitely no exception to this rule. I am curious to wonder how many times it was suggested for psychological benefits alone? I bet not many, if any at all. Plant-based foods and therapies are not only good for the body, but they're excellent for treating and balancing the mind. Within the realm of Ayurveda, plant-based modalities have been not only given the proper attention, but they have their own category and subcategories called *medhya rasayana*. Plant-based medicines are broken down into two separate categories based on their specific actions; their cognitive function or nootropic action. I must take a moment here, however, as I have many times in the past while training and educating athletes and bodybuilders, to explain that there is no substitution for whole food and proper diet and lifestyle. We have become blind to the actual definition of the term "supplement". They are not called "replacements," so they should not be used as so. Their efficacy comes into play when trying to bolster treatments and to fill nutritional voids.

I am not going to make the focus of this chapter's section on Ayurvedic herbology, but I do want to take a few moments and cover several specific herbs that are effective neurotonics. The first one that comes to mind is *ashwagandha;* withania somnifera. *Ashwagandha*, or as it is often referred to as Indian Ginseng, is a plant where the stem and the berry is utilized for medicinal purposes. It is a well-known adaptogen, and therefore can be used to help reduce the effects of stress within both the body and the mind. A 2012 study showed that after 60 days of treatment with *ashwagandha*, adults with a history of chronic stress showed a significant reduction in stress and serum cortisol levels versus the placebo group[46]. The Journal of Alternative and Complementary Medicine conducted a systematic review of all research into the herb and of the five studies that met their criteria, all five found evidence that treatment with *ashwagandha* resulted in improvements in anxiety and stress levels.

Having been used successfully for many generations in Ayurvedic traditions, *ashwagandha* is described as an herbal preparation that promotes a youthful state of physical and mental health and expands happiness. In Ayurveda this is called *Rasayanna*. This wonder hern is usually prepared as a powder and the powder can be added to a ghee, honey or even a *doshic* specific oil. It enhances the function of the brain and nervous system and improves the memory. It improves the function of the reproductive system promoting a healthy sexual and reproductive balance. Being a powerful adaptogen, it enhances the body's resilience to stress. The versatility, low cost and widescope of its efficacy makes this super-herb a go to for anyone looking to help bring the mind back into a state of balance.

As I have mentioned in one of my previous books titled, <u>Law of One Mind</u>, your thoughts are not random and fleeting things holding no power or consequences. As the famous saying goes, "thoughts become things," and the ageless philosophies of Ayurveda concur. The mind is as powerful as it's peculiar. Thoughts not only become things, but they are also nourishing.

---

[46] "A Prospective, Randomized Double-Blind, Placebo ... - NCBI." https://www.ncbi.nlm.nih.gov/pmc/articles/PMC3573577/. Accessed 7 Jan. 2020.

Thoughts are active, all-encompassing and are either fueling or destroying your current state of health. Being an advocate of good mental health, the systems brought forth by the ancient Ayurvedic traditions will help you fully utilize the powers of your mind for maintaining a balanced state of health and a life full of inner and outer riches beyond your imagination.

Pathology & Disease

"For those having exalted mind, qualities and actions the crops grew endowed with inconceivable rasa, virya, vipaka, prabhava, and other properties due to the presence of all qualities in earth."

— Charaka Samhita, Vimanasthana, Chapter 3, verse 24

अतिरंजित मन वाले लोगों के लिए, गुण और कार्य, फसलें बेमिसाल रस, कुंवारी, विपाका, प्रभा, और अन्य गुणों के साथ संपन्न होती हैं, जो पृथ्वी में सभी गुणों की उपस्थिति के कारण होती हैं।

Atiranjit man vaale logon ke lie, gun aur kaary, phasalen bemisaal ras, kunvaaree, vipaaka, prabha, aur any gunon ke saath sampann hotee hain, jo prthvee mein sabhee gunon kee upasthiti ke kaaran hotee hain.

The importance of understanding the differences between "healthcare" and "sickcare" can lead you down the path towards a deeper utilization of the true brilliance of Ayurveda. It is far easier to maintain a state of homeostasis than it is to return a body of disease to a state of ease. Not only is it straightforward and simple, but it is far less expensive. Easier and less expensive - haven't we become a society of wanting greater ease and more money? Then why is it that we neglect our health and find ourselves in a constant battle against the natural and effortless rhythms of life?

The state of your health is in constant flux, for everything in the universe follows this law. This is law... not a choice! You cannot become ignorant to it and are unable to exert human will to override it. Being woven into the underlying fabric of the universe, it works silently and continually. Nobody and nothing is outside its continual ebb and flow. By moving forward with this knowledge then it stands to reason that caring for your well-being becomes something that must constantly be appreciated. It is at this precise moment where the simplistic nature of Ayurveda becomes ever so important. You see, Ayurveda is a system that was formed based on keeping oneself in a constant state of balance. Residing in a continual state of balance yields good health, which ultimately leads to happiness and then to love. What you think, do and eat today becomes a part of who you'll be and the life you'll lead tomorrow. Just as what you see in the mirror today is a collection of what you did or did not do yesterday - and of course, the days prior.

It is amazing that even though everyone differs in their unique constitutions, we all fall victim regarless of age, race, creed or sex to even the slightest derrangement of the five universal elements; space, air, fire, water and earth. There is a universal order and flow to the derangement and balancing of the elements, therefore, any system of health needs to coincide with these indisputable laws. The care and management of the continually changing aspects of the *panchamahabhutas* (5 elements) is what you'll learn in this chapter and beyond. It clearly states in the treatise that the root cause of any disease is the "unrighteousness" of the *tridoshas*. You may be wondering, I assume, what can you do in order to stay righteous?

According to Ayurveda the pathology of disease is broken down into three causative factor: (1) Innate, meaning caused by a disturbance of the *dosha*. (2) Exogenous: caused by *bhuta* (spirits & organisms), poisoned air, fire, trauma, etc. And (3) Psychic: caused by non-fulfillment of desires and facing of the undesired[47]. It is important to understand that from here there is certainty in the causes of disorders of any of the above. They are the excessive, negative and perverted uses of sense objects, actions and time. As an example, excessive exposure to loud music will increase the air element within the neuro-physical humors, thus disturbing the *vata dosha*. Consuming too much spicy foods will create an excess of the fire element. An excess of the fire element leads to a disruption of the *pitta dosha*. A disruption of the *pitta dosha* can lead to mental or physical manifestations governed by this particular bodily humor, such as hyperacidity.

Despite the simplistic nature of these timeless traditions it is, however, a bit more involved than overindulgence or lack thereof. The holding or forces of bodily urges such as urination or sleep will cause a disturbance of the *doshas*. In short, the guidelines following the psychic and physical aggravation of the *doshas* are unsuitable contact of objects with sense organs and intellectual error. When looking at diet alone, most often the consumption and use of wholesome food promotes the growth of person, where more often than not, the consumption and use of unwholesome food is the cause of disorders. There are exceptions to this, whereas the above is not fully black and white.

---

[47] Sushruta Samhita, chapter 20 verses 3-4

Someone consuming only wholesome foods can still fall ill. When this is the case there are three suspects:

1. Abnormality in time factor

2. Intellectual error

3. Unsuitable sound, touch, vision, taste and smell

There are times, of course, and you may know someone who appears to be living an unhealthy lifestyle but doesn't seem to fall victim to disease as often as you think. There are several factors at play. One major factor being that the fault doesn't produce derangements immediately due to certain reasons such as the unwholesome aspects are not equal to the derangement itself. Secondly, there hasn't passed an adequate amount of time for the disorder to manifest on the physical plane. The important thing here to realize is that not everyone is equally capable to resist disease. The strength of one's immunity is a key factor, as is their state of mind and its corresponding thoughts. Someone who is too lean, even despite consuming mainly fruits and vegetables will be more susceptible to disease due to the imbalanced nature of their bodily humor (*vikruti*). The overconsumption of vegetables that are high in the air element such as spinach or kale is very aggravating for someone who is too lean. To observe it may appear that they're healthy and are fostering a greater state of health by eating a diet consisting of mainly raw vegetables, but let me tell you, this is not always true. How would you counterbalance a body that is too lean, too dry and too frail? Not everyone who is thin is healthy and not everyone who appears to be overweight is unhealthy.

When looking at disease it is just as important to understand how disease develops, as it is knowing how to treat an illness. At this point, it is too late, the disease has already manifested. There are an endless number of factors contributing to disease. The plentitude of factors can be internal or external. Understanding the importance of this aspect of human health, Ayurveda has brought forth 6 stages of the disease process. The unique aspect to this approach to pathology is that the first 2 stages of disease has no corresponding physical manifestations. In order to help illustrate this point, let's examine the following scenario. A 42 year-old male, let's call him Edward, walks into his doctor's office complaining that he isn't feeling well and has low energy. His doctor examines the usual and takes his temperature and weight. Finding nothing abnormal, the doctor orders further testing such as blood tests. The tests are returned showing no abnormalities, to which Edward's doctor tells him that he is fine and to get more rest. A year or so later Ed is diagnosed with Type II diabetes. This sad scenario, though only fictional, is a common occurrence within the Western model of medicine each and every day. The 6 stages of disease (*satkriyākāla*) according to Ayurveda are as follows:

1. Accumulation
2. Aggravation
3. Dissemination
4. Localization
5. Manifestation
6. Disruption or Chronicity

When looking at the above, the first two stages of disease are virtually undetectable to our modern diagnostic approaches. Even during stage three, there is very little physical manifestations, so this stage of disease is often missed and left untreated. During the first three stages of disease the opportunities for treating the imbalance are many, not to mention they're far easier and far less expensive to correct. Let's take a deeper look into the six stages of disease.

Stage One: Accumulation - In this stage one of more (often times just one's main constitution) becomes aggravated. This is the stage of the disease process where the *dosha* begins to accumulate in its natural seat or organ on the body; *vata* = colon, *pitta* = small intestine, *kapha* = stomach or chest. The disturbances are mild and are certainly detectable via Ayurvedic diagnostic modalities, such as pulse reading. As an example, the increase of mucus in the lungs is an indication of an accumulation of the *kapha dosha*. At this stage this imbalance can be treated with mostly diet and lifestyle changes.

Stage Two: Aggravation - During stage two, the qualitative nature of the accumulation transitions in a quantitative nature, meaning it begins to spill over into other seats within the same *dosha*. This is what is referred to as a "vitiation" of the bodily humors. The imbalance during this stage of disease is still easy to thwart, but as the accumulation moves into other areas it does become more complicated to treat.

Stage Three: Dissemination - Stage three is where the imbalance begins to manifest and show its ugly face, though the symptoms are mild or can be still undetectable by conventional methods. The accumulation has moved into other areas, or as they're often referred to as "second seats". During this stage, abnormal or excessive food cravings will develop. As an example, if there is a vitiation of the *kapha dosha*, one may experience a desire to eat a greater amount of sweets. Minor aches and pains can begin to be experienced during this stage. The addition of herbal remedies can be useful in treating an imbalance in this particular stage of disease.

Stage Four: Localization - In this stage the *dosha* now localizes in a tissue outside of its main seat and begins to disrupt the function of that tissue (*dhatu*) or organ. All of the *doshas* will begin to act similarly. At this stage, the accumulation will seek out the weakest part of the body and begin to manifest in that particular area. This space is called *khavaigunya* in Ayurveda[48]. Once it becomes localized it begins to disrupt the cell function of that area and this is where physical manifestation and symptoms can be detectable. During this stage of disease is where the formation of *ama* comes into play due to the fact that our digestive process is usually impaired. As an example, if the accumulation of the *kapha dosha* has spilled over into the chest and lungs you may notice an even greater increase of phlegm and mucus and could be suffering from a chest cold. Feeling heavy and lethargic will be more common physical experiences.

Stage Five: Manifestation - At the fifth stage, the localized spot becomes overwhelmed and often requires prompt medical attention. The disease can also start affecting other organs if left untreated. The function of the tissues

---

[48] "Khavaigunya - allAyurveda." 14 May. 2018, https://allayurveda.com/glossary/khavaigunya/. Accessed 13 May. 2018.

becomes impaired. This usually manifests as some sort of inflammation. This is the stage where you'll often find yourself saying, "I am sick".

Stage Six: Disruption or Chronicity - During stage six, the disease process becomes embedded into bodily tissues. This is a very serious stage of disease, whereas the body's natural defenses are not able to reverse the effects of the imbalance. The disturbance becomes long-term, chronic and in some cases, life threatening. For example, the imbalance to the *kapha dosha* could become chronic or perennial sinusitis or rhinitis. This is the hardest stage to reverse and usually requires the most comprehensive form of treatment, or multiple healing modalities.

As you can see, prevention is the key and it is during the preventative stages of the disease process where modern medicine is of little or no need. It isn't until the later or more advanced stages of disease where modern medicine and / or surgical procedures will become necessary to help reverse the effects of the disease. Once these advanced medical procedures are employed, the aid of consuming a healthy and balanced diet, as well as living a lifestyle specific to your unique constitution becomes critical. If this is not performed in accordance, the disease will return or manifest yet again as another chronic malady.

Another interesting aspect of Ayurveda's take on disease is the fact that the Ayurvedic texts strongly emphasize that it is not necessary to name every disease. The understanding of the disease in terms of *nidāna* (etiology), *dosa* (dysfunction), and *dūsya* (target tissues) as well as the stages of progress of the disease was considered to be crucial in succeeding in the treatment[49].

A foundation based upon the theory of *tridoshas* was brought forth and developed as the primary tool used to quantify the pathogenesis and consequently qualify the need for any lifestyle or medical interventions. Within the framework of this model, you will bring forth the knowledge and comprehension to make the necessary diet and lifestyle changes when and where needed, based solely upon your individual makeup (*prakruti*) and the derangement of the specific *doshas*. You'll be armed with the necessary knowledge in knowing how to correct any imbalance of the bodily humors by an easy system of employing the nature of the imbalances' opposites. This will mainly be done by making minor and suitable lifestyle changes. If the process of disease goes unnoticed or unattended and advances into further stages of the disease process, then you can feel confident knowing you'll possess the ability to perform cleansing processes such as *panchakarma or* the 5 actions to eliminate unwanted toxins and buildup of *ama*. By reversing the degradation process and restoring vitality and balance to your tissues and *dosha*, you can progress through life no longer having to live under the black cloud of becoming a helpless victim to disease.

---

[49] Murthy KRS, translator. Vaghbhata's Ashtanga Hrdayam. Varanasi: Krishnadas Academy; 1996. P. 179.

Lifestyle & Routine

"...endowed with learning and intelligence, memory, dexterity, restraint, regular use of wholesome regimen, purity of speech, serenity of mind and patience."
- Susruta Samhita, Sutra Sthana, Chapter 28, verse 36, 38

सीखने और बुद्धिमत्ता, स्मृति, निपुणता, संयम के साथ संपन्न, नियमित रूप से पौष्टिक आहार का उपयोग, भाषण की शुद्धता, मन की शांति और धैर्य

seekhane aur buddhimatta, smrti, nipunata, sanyam ke saath sampann, niyamit roop se paushtik aahaar ka upayog, bhaashan kee shuddhata, man kee shaanti aur dhairy

At our most fundamental level, our physiology is centered upon and adaptive to some sort of routine. Humans are, by their very nature, creatures of habit. This unconsciously allows us to promote health and wellness. Within the Ayurvedic point of view, as well as that of modern medicine, our daily routines are intricate to our health on many different facets. Having a balanced and structured routine, especially for the *vata dosha*, as an example, can help us regulate our sleeping patterns, reduce stress, and improve digestion and our overall eating habits. A daily routine fosters a better use of our limited time and for most, is fun and far less stressful. In effect, having a daily routine offers the grounding, stability and predictability that are largely absent from our hectic modern lives. Unlike here in the west, however, our daily routines are to be best suited to our *dosha* and to bring back an overall state of balance to the mind and body. By combining the importance of our *doshic* makeup to our daily routines, we are, as a result, eliciting profound rejuvenation throughout the body without requiring any conscious awareness of the healing process.

One of the more important aspects to creating a daily routine, outside stressing the importance of our *dosha*, is to create a manageable schedule. Developing your daily routine around tasks which you are not able to perform or are unwilling to perform, is not only a waste of time, but can induce a state of stress. Begin by incorporating those aspects that are quick and easy to manage and then progressively move onto more difficult and more unfamiliar aspects. By doing so, and prioritizing your daily activities, you are, in fact, taking control and responsibility for your health and your life. No longer will you need to, nor should you, fall victim to unlucky happenstance. Even though, of course, there is no such thing.

I was never considered to be a mathematician, and since I need to get naked to count to 21, I will not even begin to fathom the endless combinations of *doshic* possibilities. As I have previously mentioned, even despite the fact that you possess a predominance of one of the three *doshas*, we are all a unique blend of each of the *panchamahabhutas*. In addition, our minds and physical bodies can be two entirely different *doshas*. For instance, my specific *dosha* is predominantly *pitta*, but I exhibit a strong *vata* mind. It is in situations like this where managing the delicate balance and interplay between the body and mind becomes a bit trickier but nonetheless, important. The possibilities are endless, and we will look at the unique coaction between your mind and body moving forward. I will create sample daily plans for all three body-types shortly. Perhaps you'll be lucky and will fit closely into one of the examples provided. If not and you feel you need further help you can always order your reader specific version of this work. Either way, by the time you are finished reading this book, the information I have provided, coupled with the examples forthcoming, will help you to confidently move forward with a knowledge that will prepare and arm you with the tools and skills needed to live a balanced and healthy life. You will never again need to fall victim to the constant bombardment of scams and dietary disceptions lacing our personal social media platforms. Remember, until someone uncovers your unique constitution and truly understands the philosophy and science behind the principles I've covered in this work, any suggestions they provide are purely blind, unwarranted, and oftentimes dangerous.

Your True Nature & Your Daily Routine

Understanding your true nature is crucial, yes, but it is just part of the full equation. Knowing how the interplay of the bioenergetic rhythms of your physio-psychological body intertwines with the natural rhythms of the universe is of utmost importance. Believing and understanding that even the slightest excess or deficiency in any aspect of these bioenergetic rhythms results in a disturbance at the *doshic* level, becomes important. As you've just learned in the previous chapter, if any imbalance is left unattended disease will surely ensue. Even listening to your car radio at a volume that is too loud can cause an excess of the *vata dosha*. Simply knowing who you are is not enough.

If disease occurs within the vitiation of any of the three bodily humors (*doshas*), then it would stand to reason that good health can exist within the realm of a reversal of fortune. You must understand, however, that the pendulum swing between balanced and unbalanced (*prakriti* v.s. *vikriti*) is constant and continual. It is almost impossible to be residing in a state of exact. In addition, there will often be times where the needle of the pendulum may sway more towards a state of imbalance. The further the needle is allowed to swing towards a state of imbalance, the more difficult and the more serious the imbalance will manifest. This is the beauty and simplistic nature of this science; it is a system which stresses the importance of disease prevention - avoidance is always the best cure. As you'll learn in the coming chapters, the Ayurvedic treatises do extensively cover, however, curative measures. It is one of the purest forms of holistic healthcare ever established, and I am nonetheless amazed that even in today's fast-paced and extremely high tech society, it is alive and flourishing.

As you know, your given constitution was set forth at the time of your conception and though most factors are difficult to change, the sciences of today have revealed that many genetic factors can in fact be changed. Even though aspects such as your level of intelligence can be changed throughout the course of your life, your *prakriti* holds true and is steadfast. If, for example, you would prefer to be more *kapha dosha* (earth & water elements) in order to gain greater muscularity for the up and coming Mr. Olympia contest, you cannot...it simply doesn't work that way. Sure, there are several things you can do in order to create a greater muscular physique, but you cannot switch or swap your God-given constitution. Any attempts towards doing so only creates an excess of that *dosha*, and if not return to a balanced state, disease will be the result. You will soon learn to accept the beauty of your true nature and will discover how to thrive in accordance with your inherent mental, emotional and physical traits. In doing so, you'll be able to harness your natural tendencies and will flourish in all areas of life and love.

One very important aspect of Ayurveda is Ontology and Theory. Ontology, as you know, is a systematic account of existence. There are 4 major ways of "knowing," according to the ancient Ayurvedic texts. They are as follows:

1. Knowledge gained from individuals who have foregone material needs
2. Through personal observation
3. Through experimentation
4. Logical conclusion from observed phenomena[50]

The principles of Ayurveda are mostly holistic in their nature and in their methodology. The approach of Ayurveda is comprised of an epistemology that varies quite differently from the modern approach to biomedicine, which is far more reductionist in its methods. By understanding and coming in tune with nature, Ayurveda has theorized a system utilizing the natural rhythms of the universe in order to create harmony within our minds, bodies and spirits. Unlike the pharmaceutical approach which is based solely upon a singular

---

[50] "Ayurveda research: Ontological challenges - NCBI." https://www.ncbi.nlm.nih.gov/pmc/articles/PMC3326789/. Accessed 12 May. 2018.

chemical compound designed to affect a single organ, tissue or anomalies, the holistic approach takes into consideration the whole being; meaning holistic. Within the realm of Ayurveda, you cannot selectively heal; you cannot correct gout and ignore fibromyalgia. You cannot improve your digestion without positively affecting your entire system, both physically and mentally. Likewise, you cannot create an imbalance anywhere within the mind and body that does not negatively affect the whole. Viewing the body and its many systems as individual entities working separately is wrong...in every sense of the imagination. It is viewed that everything in the universe is both a medicine and a poison; medicine if utilized properly and poison if used improperly.

In Ayurveda, they not only stress the importance of living a specific, proper and balanced lifestyle, they also provide the knowledge and means of experiencing that exact existence. In Ayurveda, this is called *dinacharya*, as mentioned earlier. In addition to the six tastes and their relationship to diet, exercise and seasonality, personal hygiene is also stressed. The body is a temple, a living vessel, and proper maintenance and growth is essential to the overall well-being of the organism. It is also emphasized that one should never suppress natural physiological urges, such as urination, defecation, sneezing, yawning, hunger, thirst, sleep and even lacrimation. In the same token, the proper releasing of negative emotions and urges is strongly recommended, not only within the boundaries of the Ayurvedic text, but it is also urged in western medicine. Many of today's top cardiologists, neurologists and psychiatrists are advocates for the proper diagnosis, management and processing of stress and other negative emotions, which if left unattended, can cause a slew of mental and thus physiological disturbances.

Through the means of another important principle in Ayurveda, called *swasthavritta*, preventative measures for aging and neurological decline are important components which need to be considered and blended into your daily routine. Methods employed here will include herbal remedies, proper diet, as well as exercise and mediation. You see, to the ancient Seers and Yogis the birth of mankind is not accidental or mere happenstance, but rather a meaningful journey of inner discovery. Our bodies, our minds and the blessings of this reality is but a vessel through which this discovery and union is to manifest. I liken this to a cross country road trip; you'll want to choose wisely the vehicle of your choice. A vehicle that is performing within its optimal capacity, of course, is the best choice. The same goes for our minds and bodies; a healthy vessel is a happy vessel through which man will enjoy and experience the greatest journeys of life. Never was there a great experience ever lived while one was sick and dying in bed. Disease-free living and a daily maintenance is but the only true way for one to maintain a perfect state of mind and body.

The Vata Daily Routine

"Tatra ruksho laghu sheetah, khara sukshmaschalo nilah:
the qualities of Vata are dry, light, cool, rough, subtle & Mobile."

- **Ashtanga Hrdayam: Sutrasthana 1:11**

वात के गुण शुष्क, हल्के, शांत, खुरदरे, सूक्ष्म और मोबाइल हैं

Universal Elements - Space and Air
Pacifying Tastes - Sweet and Pungent
Aggravating Tastes - Bitter and Astringent
Pacifying Season - Summer and Spring
Aggravating Season -Fall and Winter

Natural Qualities & Physical Characteristics:

- Slender and thin, difficulty in gaining weight
- Height is taller or shorter than average
- Thin hair
- Energy fluctuates and comes in bursts
- Appetite is variable
- Tendency towards constipation or dry stool
- Dry skin, hair and nails; Nails are often fragile
- Light sleeper, erratic sleeping patterns and often suffers from insomnia

- Prefers warmer and moist weather

Psychological Characteristics:

- Creative and imaginative
- Artistic
- Active and restless
- Quick learner, difficulty in remembering
- Becomes 'spaced-out' quite easily
- Tendency to feel anxious, nervous and insecure
- Speaks quickly and often uses hand gestures
- Difficulty in staying still or sitting for long periods of time
- Irregular routine
- Experiences colorful dreams

Famous Vata Person: Mick Jagger

Signs & Symptoms of an Air & Space Vitiation

There are many indicators of an increase of the air and space elements, especially those causing a mental or physical manifestation. Any given mental or physical manifestation can reside as an increase or decrease of any of the *doshas*, but normally certain symptoms and imbalances will primarily indicate an increase or decrease of a specific universal element. Here is a brief list of common signs of a *vata* imbalance (this is just a partial list and *vata* imbalances are not limited to the below):

- Excessive worry
- Fatigue and poor stamina
- Nervousness, difficulty in concentrating
- Anxious and fearful
- Impatient and hyperactive
- Insecure and shy
- Indecisiveness
- Underweight
- Insomnia
- Sensitive to cold weather
- Fainting spells
- Irregular heartbeat or palpitations
- Dry, rough or chapped skin and/or lips
- Joint pain or excessive joint discomfort
- Constipation, bloating or excessive gas

Living their lives based upon erratic and unpredictable behavior is something which the *vata* person yearns for, or at least, doesn't mind. This is an aspect of their true nature driven by the energetic bio-rhythms of the universe and its corresponding elements. You can never guess their next move, and move they surely will. Embrace your wandering nature, it is a part of who you are.

Treating disease, creating a lifestyle plan and deciding what occupation to choose requires a thought process based around your inherent nature. If you are suffering from a disease due to an increase of the air and/or space elements, than your daily routine must reflect its opposite nature. Living in accordance with your God-given *dosha* sets the stage for not only living in a state of balance, but will allow you to thrive in a career field that best compliments your natural traits. Remember, like creates more of the like; opposite creates balance. By choosing certain aspects of your daily routine, you will allow the true nature of air and space to shine through brilliantly in all you do.

One important distinction I must mention here, is just because a food or activity or whatnot may fall on the "do not consume" list, does not mean that they always need to be fully avoided. Moderation and being mindful are two critical components when you find yourself compelled to indulge in something that may not be pacifying to your light and airy nature. Where you need to be the most disciplined, however, is when you're suffering from any digestive disturbance or are experiencing any other mental or physical ailment. Symptoms are merely whispers something is wrong. Never allow yourself to witness their violent screams!

Hyperactivity is a common *vata* trait, so eating 3 meals a day at preferably the same times becomes an easy, yet important distinction. By doing so you'll unconsciously create a routine, and routines for the airy and spacy type is just what the doctor ordered - most days. Engaging in erratic behaviors, erratic eating habits or eating on the move is a definite no-no! Yes, this may seem at the moment to be a daunting task, but small steps results in major changes. Since dusk is the end of the *vata* time period, eating heavier, but easy to digest foods at dinner is advisable. Lunch should be your biggest meal of the day, followed by dinner and then breakfast. The amount as well as the physiological effect of your ingredients needs to always be taken into consideration. As an example, even though breakfast should be the smallest and easiest to digest meal, it also should be grounding. An avocado omelette, with a pinch of sea salt and black pepper would be a great choice given the proper time of year. And I am sorry to say, snacking and frequent meals are off limits.

The sweet taste pacifies *vata* the most, however, you need to understand that I am not giving you a prescription to eat sugary and highly processed treats. Foods that are naturally sweet, like beets and carrots are what I am referring to. Even meats, if you are comfortable consuming them and assuming your digestive state is working optimally, are okay in moderation. Most grains, especially wheat, is also sweet. Avoidance of sugary foods that provide a temporary quick boost of energy followed by a crash should be avoided at all times. If you're a coffee drinker and you're *vata*, try adding some organic grass-fed butter, organic coconut oil or ghee with a pinch of cinnamon to each cup. This is a great way to increase your metabolism, as well as incorporate healthy fats into your diet. These healthier fats can help lubricate joints, hair, skin and nails that may be dry and brittle. Sounds weird, I know, but try it!

The importance of understanding the art of eating will be a crucial component of your customized plan. Below I will provide sample meal plans for the *tridoshas* that you may use as a starting point and as a general guideline. As a reminder, your geographic location and the current season does play a significant level of importance when creating, executing and monitoring any meal or lifestyle plan. Without knowing these, as well as other specifics, the guidelines below can be nothing other than recommendations. Any positive step, however, can initiate both short term and long term results of a similar nature. No step is too small and no change will be considered insignificant moving forward. Here is a list of foods that the *vata* type will want to avoid or eliminate. Again, this can only be a partial and generalized list and certainly doesn't apply to everyone.

Vata Aggravating Foods

- Most leafy greens such as kale, arugula and spinach
- Cabbages
- Bitter greens
- Dry legumes
- Rough and stale foods
- Most beans
- Popcorn
- Dried fruits
- Raw vegetables
- Refined sugars
- Leftovers
- Carbonated drinks

- Hollow vegetables with seeds, except bell peppers, especially the spicier more pungent peppers

Vata Pacifying Foods

- Most fruits, especially avocado and banana
- Most grains like oatmeal and basmati rice
- Most meats, especially seafood
- Red lentils, split yellow mung beans
- Most dairy products like butter, ghee, cream, whole milk (warmed, whereas warmed dairy products are much easier to digest)
- Most root vegetables like carrots, beets, turnips, celery root, eggplant, pumpkin / squash, sweet potatoes, white potato is okay in moderation

Vata Pacifying Spices & Herbs

- Black pepper & red pepper
- Ginger
- Nutmeg
- Cardamom
- Cinnamon
- Clove
- Coriander
- Fennel
- Mustard seed

- Rock salt or sea salt
- Garlic

To better help you understand the premise of why a food is or isn't balancing I will break down a few of the above foods in greater detail.

Kale - the qualities of kale are cold, dry and light. The taste of kale is bitter and astringent, all of which are aggravating to the *vata dosha* due to their inherent capacity for air and space.

Beans - the qualities of most beans (green beans are the exception here) are dry and difficult to digest. If you must consume beans, soak them overnight before preparing them, and cook them slowly and thoroughly. Most beans are astringent in taste, thus rendering them an overall bad choice for the *vata dosha* or someone exhibiting an excess of the air and space elements.

Avocado - the qualities of avocados are gooey, oily, heavy and easy. All of these qualities are consistent with an opposite nature to the elemental aspect of the *vata dosha*, making them excellent choices. The taste of the avocado is sweet, and sweet if you recall is comprised of earth and water; both of a balancing nature to air and space.

Cinnamon - the qualities of cinnamon are dry, light, easy and hot. So in essence, cinnamon has a warming and drying effect upon the body and the mind. The taste of cinnamon is sweet, pungent and slightly astringent.

Moreover it has a warming effect and astringent quality; this is a spice that even despite the fact that is can be balancing for *vata dosha*, they need to use in moderation.

Vata Sample Daily Routine

Awaken: 6:00 a.m.
Clean Teeth & Mouth: 6:15 a.m.
Consume Warm Water & Lemon: a few minutes following the cleaning of your teeth and mouth
Yoga or Meditation: 7:00 a.m.
Bathe & Self-Oil Treatment (*abhyanga*): 7:30 a.m.
Breakfast (1st meal of the day): 8:00 a.m.
Lunch (2nd meal of the day): Noontime
Dinner (3rd meal of the day): 6:00 p.m.
Bedtime: 10:00 p.m. - sleep on your left side or back (barring injury)

It is important to remember here that the above are suggestions and often life is at times very unpredictable. As an example, if you are required to attend a morning meeting at 7:00 a.m. which is unusual, of course, you will not want to inform your boss you won't attend because it interferes with your morning *abhyanga*. Together we will make strides to change what needs to be changed and deal with what we cannot as we proceed.

The *vata dosha* can opt to take a quick, warm shower or bath prior to exercise. Doing so will help alleviate any stiff and tense muscles, as well as increase blood flow. If time or conditions do not allow for a warming shower or bath, then properly warming up becomes one of the more critical aspects of your exercise routine.

Vata Sample Meal Plan - Autumn

Breakfast:

warm oatmeal with whole milk or ghee,

seasoned with cinnamon, nutmeg and a pinch of rock salt

or

sliced tomato and avocado

seasoned with rock salt and black pepper

with

spiced chai tea

Lunch:

vegetable or lentil soup (slightly pungent)

or

sauteed carrots, onions, bell peppers, garlic and ginger

with ghee over a bed of quinoa

with

warm water or ginger tea

Dinner:

baked sweet potato with ghee

or

mung dal kitchari

with

warm water of ginger tea

As the colder months come to an end and your body is no longer in a building and storage mode, you need to shift your focus to that of renew and release. To the delight of most, your body will naturally want to shed some of the extra weight it had accumulated over the winter months. Changing your diet and your daily routine becomes just as important, if not more important, than changing your wardrobes. Transitioning from winter into the warmer months of spring, is one of the most important times of the year to perform a detox. Doing so releases the excess stagnation of the blood, tissues and various organs of the body.

The diet, exercise and daily routines of the *vata* individual needs to be grounding and nourishing. Those who exhibit higher levels of the air and space elements make naturally good runners, especially long distances. The key here is developing a means of cultivating their natural tendencies and to successfully meld it with more grounding movements and foods. Yoga is an excellent way to ground the active mind of the *vata* type, as well as help keep the tendons and muscles flexible and lubricated, especially during physical exercise. A slightly more meditative style yoga, approximately 2-3 times a week is recommended. We will get more into yoga and its benefits and relation to Ayurveda in a coming chapter.

By focusing on your natural abilities and what you enjoy the most, you create a way of living rather than falling into the cruel reality of a specific diet or exercise routine. As an example and as I've just mentioned above, the *vata* person will normally love to run - and run they should. They need to be cautious, however, if ever experiencing an elevation of this particular *dosha* and during the windier and drier months of fall. Your body changes daily...the weather and our environment changes just as often. With this in mind, if during the fall you experience a warmer and moist day, then yes, you can enjoy a longer and more vigorous run. Being mindful of your body, its current state, your food and your immediate environment is a skill that we all need to learn, understand incorporate each and every day.

Sample Exercise Routine - Vata

If you're the *vata* type and are looking or are needing to gain greater muscle mass and strength, than I recommend a two-day split routine focused are hypertrophy . Below is a sample hypertrophy routine for the *vata dosha*:

Monday - Lower Body
Tuesday - Yoga
Wednesday - Rest
Thursday - Upper Body
Friday - Yoga

Saturday - Strength & Endurance
Sunday - Rest

Your geographic area and the climatic conditions in which you reside plays a crucial role in the formation of your diet, exercise and overall lifestyle routines. The *vata* type, since their nature is composed of irregularity due to the nature of the space and air elements, should choose to reside in areas which offer more warmth and moisture. Two examples would be Miami or Atlanta. Phoenix, though it is one of the warmest cities in the country, may be too extreme and too dry for the *vata* type individual. The fall and winters months of these two areas are mild and offer climatic solace to the *vata* type. Also, the severity of their seasonal changes are far less than those of New York City and Boston. The *vata* type will welcome the change more than most, however, in keeping with the philosophy of like-increases-like, they need to avoid these type areas if possible. If not, and moving or relocating is not an option, you will need to place an even greater importance on each and every aspect of your daily routine. In this situation there is far less room for you to err. We will look at your unique situation in your customized version of this work.

In Ayurveda, the importance of a daily routine is an aspect that is focused upon greatly. For the *vata* individual, routines cannot be stressed enough. It sets the stage for the entire day, helps to eliminate undue stress and anxiety, as well as produces a calming and grounding effect upon your mind and your body. Consuming regular meals and exercising at the same time of day is something you will need to effectively incorporate into your new lifestyle.

Even waking up and grooming at similar times is important and keeps the airy-type focused and better grounded. By observing and understanding the rhythm of nature, you can be in better tune with both the ebb and flow around you, as well as your ever-changing internal environment. Disease prevention is an age-old Ayurvedic adage. It is achieved by consciously making small daily choices to keep you in alignment with your natural tendencies. The beauty and simplicity of this Vedic science is understanding—in any given moment—what will help you bring about alignment. As we age and change naturally, every aspect of your daily routine will need to change. Remember, as humans we live and reside within a state of being that is constantly evolving - a reality of generation, degeneration and regeneration. You cannot escape this, as I am sure many over the ages have tried. No longer should you need to worry and fight this, but rather live in gracious harmony with nature and its governing laws.

The Pitta Daily Routine

"Pittam sasneha tikshnosham laghu visram, saram dravam."
Pitta is oily, sharp, hot, light, fleshy-smelling, spreading and liquid.

- Ashtanga Hrdayam: Sutrasthana 1:11

पित्त तैलीय, तीक्ष्ण, गर्म, हल्का, मांसल-महक, फैलने वाला और तरल होता है।

Universal Elements - Fire and Water
Pacifying Tastes - Sweet and Sour
Aggravating Tastes - Pungent and Salty
Pacifying Season - Winter and Fall
Aggravating Season - Summer and Spring

Natural Qualities & Physical Characteristics:

- Medium build, good musculature
- Average height
- Pointed features
- High energy levels
- Strong appetite, often robust
- Regular bowel movements, with a tendency towards diarrhea
- Oily skin. Reddish hue and burns easily
- Perspires easily
- Prefers cooler weather. May become irritable in warmer climates
- Penetrating eyes

Psychological Characteristics:

- Goal Oriented
- Good Sense of humor
- Strong intellect, yearns to learn
- Natural ability to read
- Critical of self and others
- Perfectionist
- Tendency towards anger and irritability, especially if a meal is skipped
- Stubborn, bull-headed
- Loves competition

Famous Pitta Person: Jennifer Aniston

Signs & Symptoms of a Fire & Water Vitiation

- Anger & irritability
- Hostile & destructive
- Impatient
- Critical of self and of others
- Argumentative & aggressive
- Controlling behavior
- Reckless in nature
- Heartburn, increased stomach acidity
- Diarrhea

- Increased food sensitivities
- Skin issues; rashed, eruptions, boils and acne
- Bad breath
- Increased body odor
- Overly sensitive to heat and light
- Hypoglycemic
- Fever and night sweats

Pitta dosha, since it is primarily formed from the fire element, is hot and spicy. The energetic properties of *pitta* are in a constant state of transformation. This fire within you regulates digestion, all sensory inputs, your body temperature and the health and tonality of your skin. When *pitta* is experiencing a vitiation, a common imbalance can be anger and various skin disturbances. One of the main goals of someone with predominantly a *pitta* constitution is to cool it down, so to speak. As the spring ends and we quickly enter into the warmth and humid months of summer, staying cool and hydrated becomes one goal that you'll need to place an even greater emphasis.

Pittas love and thrive within the excitement of challenges and competition. They love to win and they love to compete. And though they're not in love with the steadiness of their daily routines as the *kapha* type, they enjoy a comfortable routine far more that the erratic nature of the *vata* type. I stressed in an earlier chapter the importance of not consuming foods when residing in a state of fear or anger or any of the like. This is even more important for the fiery demeanor of the *pitta*. You will focus on smaller and more cooling foods providing an adequate amount of proteins. Never fill your stomach with cold liquids prior to eating, and your last meal of the day should be at least 3 hours prior to bedtime. Oh, and only eat when you're hungry.

Other things you'll need to focus on avoiding are common culprits like too much caffeine, alcohol and salt. These are things that will increase heat and can easily cause a vitiation of the *pitta dosha*, thus manifesting as aggressive behavior and bouts of anger, not to mention a slew of physiological issues. Here is a short list of foods that will cause an increase of the *pitta dosha*:

Pitta Aggravating Foods

- Cayenne pepper
- Black pepper (for taste small amounts can be used)
- Salty foods
- Spinach
- Hollow vegetables with seeds, especially all pungent peppers
- Garlic
- Tomatoes
- Peanuts
- Raishes
- Refined sugars
- Rough and stale foods
- Leftovers

Pitta Pacifying Foods

- Most fruits, especially mango and watermelon
- Most grains such as oatmeal and basmati rice
- Most meats, limit seafood
- Red lentils, split yellow mung beans
- All sweet and bitter vegetables
- Almonds, coconut, pumpkin and sunflower seeds
- Most root vegetables like celery, cucumber, broccoli, leafy greens, sweet potato, pumpkin, squash and zucchini
- Most dairy products like butter, ghee, cream, cottage cheese and whole milk

Pitta Pacifying Spices

- Cardamom
- Cilantro
- Ginger
- Dill
- Coriander
- Saffron
- Turmeric (in smaller amounts, can be heating in overconsumption)
- Mints
- Hing

To further your understanding into the nature of the foods you eat and their inherent qualities, I will explain and break down a few foods from the above list and break them down for you. Knowing this and understanding how delicate their interplay is with your health is something I cannot stress nearly enough.

Garlic - the qualities (*guna*) of garlic are hot and clear. Its taste is pungent. Pungency is mainly comprised of the fire element, thus, even despite its many touted health benefits, makes it an unwise choice for then *pitta dosha* - especially during the summer months.

Tomato - the quality (*guna*) of tomatoes is difficult. Its tastes are sweet, sour and pungent, making it pacifying for *vata* and aggravating for *kapha* and *pitta*. In the summertime, raw tomatoes can have a cooling effect upon blood, hence, in smaller amounts making it a rare exception for the *pitta dosha*.

Cardamom - its qualities (*guna*) are mobile, light, clear and dry. Its taste is pungent, however, making it one of the few foods that is balancing in the appropriate amounts to all *doshas*. Cardamom is a natural muscle relaxant, making it a good choice after strenuous summer activities and workouts.

One aspect of your daily routine stressed through the ancient Ayurvedic texts is the importance placed upon the early hours of the morning, most of which, are the moments from when you awaken to when you consume your first meal. A greater opportunity for obtaining peace and tranquility exists within the early hours of the morning which embodies an inherent stillness. This is a great time to indulge in reflective practices and self-care. We will place an importance upon your morning practices as we progress through the process of creating your perfect daily routine.

Pitta Sample Daily Routine

Awaken: 5:30 a.m.
Clean Teeth & Mouth: 5:45 a.m.
Consume Warm Water: a few minutes following the cleaning of your teeth and mouth
Yoga or Meditation: 6:00 a.m.
Bathe & Self-Oil Treatment (*abhyanga*): 6:30 a.m.
Breakfast (1st meal of the day): 7:30 a.m.
Lunch (2nd meal of the day): Noontime
Dinner (3rd meal of the day): 6:00 p.m.
Bedtime: 10:00 p.m. - sleep on your right side or back (barring injury)

Sample Pitta Meal Plan - Summer

Breakfast:

roasted coconut flaxseed oatmeal with whole milk or coconut milk, seasoned with cinnamon, nutmeg and a pinch of rock salt

or

homemade apple sauce w/ ginger and ghee
seasoned with rock salt and black pepper

with

mint green tea

Lunch:

carrot soup with sesame seeds and raisins, sprinkled with coriander

or

sauteed kale with sweet potato and ginger

with

warm water & lemon or mint green tea

Dinner:

salmon burger

or

mung dal kitchari

with

warm water or mint green tea

Sample Exercise Routine - Pitta

Like the *pitta* pacifying diet, the exercise routine for the *pitta dosha* will be specific and cooling in nature. The person who exhibits a higher amount of the fire and water element will naturally excel at competitive sports that match their personal interests. They are typically lean and muscular and will have a more difficult time building size than the *kapha* type. Balancing the fiery nature of the *pitta* individual is something which needs to be apparent in every facet of your daily routine. Water sports, yoga and skiing are excellent exercise options for this individual. Taking a more meditative approach to yoga is wise during the times where your demeanor seems more aggressive and fiery in nature. This may seem obvious, but please avoid hot yoga classes.

Swimming is one of the best exercises for the *pitta* type, especially during the summer. The cooling nature of the water not only has a balancing effect, it can also offer a calming experience. Like all aspects of our lives, there are certain times of day and year where even the *pitta* will need to limit or avoid swimming altogether. Midday during the long and hot months of the summer, it is advised to avoid excess sun exposure. This includes swimming. Swimming in the salty water of the ocean, especially during the summer months can cause an excess of the fire element. Opt for later evening swims in pools, or even better, lakes. This author is not a fan of soaking in chlorine-based pools and or tubs!

Since the physique of the *pitta* type is tone and muscular, I recommend a 4-day split resistance training routine, if, of course, increasing your overall muscle mass is one of your goals. A routine consisting of push and pull movements will be wise choices. With a split routine consisting of push and pull movements, you'll be able to incorporate aerobic exercise and other *pitta* balancing sports on your rest days. Here is a sample exercise routine:

Monday - Chest & Biceps
Tuesday - Yoga
Wednesday - Back & Triceps
Thursday - Rest

Friday - Shoulders
Saturday - Legs & Abs
Sunday - Rest

Pay attention to how you're feeling and listen to your body. What I offer are guides and mere suggestions. What you are feeling and what your own body is saying trumps all I or anyone will ever be able to tell you. Your body pays you the greatest attention, why not return the favor and listen when it is trying to tell you something. Your bodies will tell us when something that we are doing or not doing is wrong. The human body, will however, also tell us when what we are doing or not doing is right. It is a feeling of lightness and inner elation. It promotes joy and true happiness. Of course, our modern day medical establishment wants you to listen to them, not your body. Why? Simple, they are well aware of the fact that true knowledge and wisdom can only come from within, never from without. The respect and admiration I have developed over the years for the science and philosophy of Ayurveda was cultivated upon that fact that it was fostered from within and developed hand-in-hand with the Divine. The ancient Seers and Yogis drew upon inner enlightenment to form the basis of which I have penned this work for you.

Symptoms are the language of the body. Symptoms only develop when the disease has begun to manifest and progress, and it is your body's way of telling you that something is wrong. The precise manner of where you are not acting in alignment with your true nature is the exact place where you'll be guided in correcting the disorder. Masking or relieving symptoms never produces positive and long-term results and success. Sure, taking an over-the-counter pain medication for a headache will offer temporary relief. You must ask yourself, however, what is the root cause of that headache? A vitiation of the *tridoshas* is always the root cause. It is here where you'll learn to look. Now, do not misunderstand what I am saying; allowing yourself relief from aggravating or painful symptoms is a good thing. Never stop there. Let's continue on together and reveal the true source of the imbalance. That, in my book, is a win-win. And, well, this is my book...

Sometimes we do not have a choice; the tides of destiny or the rigors of your personal responsibilities can be unrelenting making living in your perfect place, working your perfect job and eating perfect foods very difficult or even impossible at certain times. Make the needed changes when or where they are available. Build upon those positive modifications and good fortune in other areas will soon follow. If you are predominantly *pitta* and live in Atlanta and are unable to move, do not fear! Changes to your diet and to other aspects of your lifestyle will help counteract the heat and humidity of your geographic area. Living in an area that is not best suited to your body-type and practicing other actions not in alignment with your *dosha* breeds imbalance. Imbalances create negative manifestations. Left unattended, these negative manifestations produce disease. Disease left unattended can produce... I think you get the picture.

The Kapha Daily Routine

"Snigdhah shita gurumandah shlakshno mritsnah sthirah kaphah"
Kapha is unctuous, cool, heavy, slow, smooth, soft and static.

- **Ashtanga Hrdayam: Sutrasthana 1:12**

काँपा अक्षत, शांत, भारी, धीमी, चिकनी, मुलायम और स्थिर होती है

Universal Elements - Earth and Water
Pacifying Tastes - Bitter and Astringent
Aggravating Tastes - Sweet and Sour
Pacifying Season - Summer and Fall (in most locations)
Aggravating Season - Winter and Spring

Natural Qualities & Physical Characteristics:

- Gains weight easily; Difficulty in losing weight
- Tendency towards obesity
- Short & stocky or tall & sturdy
- Thick hair, skin and nails
- Excellent strength and stamina
- Weak digestion, often feels heavy after eating
- Regular bowel movements
- Oily skin, that is smooth and often pale
- Sleeps easily and soundly; Tendency towards excessive sleep
- Often feels cold. Become irritable in cold and damp climates

- Prefers hot weather

Psychological Characteristics:
- Loving, calm and compassionate
- Prefers slower and easy routines and lifestyle
- Slow learner
- Exhibits a tendency towards excellent memory and retention
- Sentimental, often thinks of the past
- Protective of self and family
- Allows negative emotions to build rather than addressing them
- Prefers others take the lead, great followers
- Natural listener
- Instills trust and confidence in others

Famous Kapha Person: Shaquille O'Neal

Signs & Symptoms of a Water & Earth Vitiation

- Sluggish & dull
- Mental fog & slow cognition
- Apathetic
- Depressed, sad and overly sentimental
- Lethargic
- Procrastination
- Clingy
- Possessive

- Excessive sleep, or always tired
- Increased weight gain
- Drowsy
- Increased mucus in the throat, lungs or sinuses
- Nausea
- Pale, cold and clammy skin
- Edema, or achy and swollen joints
- Constipation, excessive gassiness or bloating

I cannot recall a day of weight training where I was not wishing I was *kapha dosha* rather than the fiery *pitta* type. Your natural strength, endurance and ability to gain muscle mass is unmatched. Having a thick and muscular physique like Arnold is not in my future. It can be, however, in the future of any *kapha* type who wishes to become the next Mr. Olympia.

Not only is your strength and natural endurance superior, you normally showcase smooth and thick skin, as well as big beautiful eyes and thick hair. Like all *doshas*, your individuality still becomes the most important aspect and last word in all decisions regarding your overall health and wellness. Just because you're *kapha dosha* doesn't mean you will become a pro-bodybuilder, nor does it guarantee you will have beautifully thick and healthy hair. Processing a greater tendency does not produce an automatic condition or state.

When suffering from an excess of the earth and water elements, the *kapha* type may suffer from excessive weight gain or even experience obesity. If you're *kapha*, you typically exhibit a slower and more sluggish digestion, which will need to be a focal point of your daily lifestyle. By exhibiting a slow and sluggish demeanor, incorporating healthy ways to get up and get moving becomes ever so important. I witness this behavior daily at the gym; heavy sets with slow deliberate movements and long rest periods. The *kapha dosha* is less subtle than the other two body-types and they're often hard to miss. The earth and water elements provide structure and lubrication to the body, so the *kapha* type will normally exhibit large joints, hair, skin and nails which demonstrates these qualities.

The main lifestyle goal of the *kapha dosha* is to get moving! Inactivity creates an atmosphere for increased lethargy, thus creating an increase of the earth and water elements. If you're *kapha* you love meat and dairy products, especially cheese and chocolate (and I am not referring to cacao, which is naturally bitter). The sweet taste, as you now are aware, is comprised of the earth and water elements. Creating a diet focused around balancing these two elements will become a focal point for the *kapha dosha*. The sour taste is aggravating, so consuming spicier and drier foods becomes important as we delve into your custom meal plan. Since the *kapha dosha* will be naturally drawn to the sweet and sour tastes, finding healthy and creative ways to incorporate the pungent and bitter taste is often a challenge. By experiencing a greater tendency towards phlegm and excess mucus, the dry and hot elements of more pungent and bitter foods will help burn off and alleviate any excess phlegm or mucus you may be experiencing.

Salads, although mostly bitter in their composition, can create a problem for the slower and more sluggish digestion of the *kapha* type. Raw veggies, in general, can be difficult to digest. As we age most experience a decline in their digestive abilities, hence, why Sophia from the Golden Girls mentioned on one particular episode to never feed her raw vegetables. Veggies that have been slightly sauteed or steamed are far better choices. Most leafy greens can be consumed raw, as they're easier to digest than vegetables such as raw carrot, broccoli and beets. Soups and kitcharis are among a few of the better dishes for the *kapha* type individual. By focusing on restoring and fostering a robust digestion, excess weight gain and digestive issues like constipation will soon become a thing of the past. Harboring a strong digestion is more important than what foods are actually being consumed. How you prepare your food is an aspect of digestion that should be addressed for all, especially those with a tendency towards slower and sluggish digestion. Highly processed food, leftovers and foods that have been microwaved or overcooked are not recommended at any time. Trying to preserve the foods' inherent properties which naturally allow for greater digestion and absorption are components of our diets that certainly need to be addressed. Raw juices, foods lightly steamed or sauteed are just a few ways that the *kapha dosha* will want to prepare their meals.

The creative incorporation of *kapha* balancing spices can be a healthy and welcomed addition. A dash of cayenne pepper or cumin can make more of a positive impact than you're probably aware, even at this point. Dancing with the natural rhythms of nature is a partner we should all choose, especially someone suffering from impaired digestion. When the sun is the highest in the sky, digestion in the human body is also at its highest. Lunchtime, hence, becomes the time of day where the *kapha* individual will want to consume their largest meal, or the meal that is the most difficult to digest; all meats and dairy will want to be consumed at this time of day. This rule is true for all, not just the *kapha dosha*, but if you are this *doshic*-type, then it becomes even more important.

The slower and often welcomed paced days of winter are seemingly a time for reflection. The calm and colder months of the winter, though offering solace for the fiery natured *pitta*, can for some begin to create excess in the water and earth elements, thus manifesting as an imbalance of the *doshas*. Every season has its inherent ability to create both order and disorder within the human body and mind. The colder, wet and damp months of the winter is certainly no exception to this rule, and is the time of year where the *kapha* type needs to be the most disciplined. For the *pitta* type, like myself, the summer becomes our critical season. Fall is the danger zone for the *vata* type.

Like increases like, yes, but opposites should attract. With this in mind, seasonality is a lifestyle component that is just as important as what you're eating. If you loathe the bitter cold days of winter, then this is the season where being precise in every aspect of your routine becomes even more important. Now, of course, not every geographic location during the winter months will feature bitter cold and wetness, which usually comes in the form of freezing rain and or snow. If winter in your area is a bit cooler and far less moist, then winter quickly becomes the time of year which could in fact more so aggravate the *vata dosha*. The more important aspect is not the name of the season itself, but rather its climatic conditions and qualities. Like all which exists in this universe, our climate is ever-changing, seamlessly swinging from one end of the pendulum to the next, even daily. Winter, ironically, due to your body naturally increasing and storing heat, is the season where your digestive fire will burn the brightest.

Kapha Aggravating Foods

- Sweet potato
- Cucumber
- Tomato
- Zucchini
- Avocado
- Banana
- Coconut
- Dates
- Grapes, melons & oranges
- Wheat (and limit rice and oat consumption)
- Most dairy products (very few exceptions)

- Leftovers
- Refined sugars
- Carbonated drinks
- Most oils, except sesame seed oil
- Most meats & animal products (some seafood is okay in smaller amounts due to higher salt content)

Kapha Pacifying Foods

- Pungent spices such as black & red pepper, clove, cinnamon & cumin
- Grains such as barley, corn, buckwheat and millet
- Cranberry, cherry, apple, pears, pomegranates, peaches and prunes
- Garlic, onion and ginger
- All beans and legumes are acceptable, except kidney beans and tofu
- Honey and pure stevia are the only acceptable sweeteners
- Sesame seeds, sunflower seeds and pumpkin seeds
- Most leafy greens such as kale, swiss chard, dandelion greens, spinach (in moderation), radishes, celery, and cauliflower

Kapha Balancing Spices

- Cardamom
- Black pepper, red pepper, chili pepper and cayenne pepper
- Fennel
- Coriander
- Saffron

- Turmeric

Let's take a moment in order to break down a few of the above. Remember, increased knowledge fosters more intelligent choices. Intelligent choices creates balance and harmony; which creates peace and happiness.

Red Meat - the qualities (*guna*) of red meats are oily, heavy, liquid and difficult. Most red meats are sweet and the sweet taste is comprised of water and earth.

Banana - the qualities (*guna*) of bananas are heavy, gooey, easy and liquid. Their taste is mainly sweet and they are very nourishing and grounding. The *kapha* type is already grounded, so consuming foods that have a natural grounding tendency can create lethargy and excess stagnation.

Black Pepper - the qualities (*guna*) of black pepper are light, hot, easy and clear. Most pepper is pungent, thus making their natural composition high in the fire element. Most forms of pepper are excellent choices for the *kapha dosha*. Now, with this said, there are several peppers that are too intense for most to handle. The habanero and ghost peppers need to be avoided, even for the *kapha dosha*.

Honey - the qualities (*guna*) of honey are clear, hot, light and dry. Surprisingly, gooey is not a quality of honey. Remember, I mentioned back in chapter one that I am not always referring to the common meaning of the word, and am often times referring to them on a subtler, more energetic level.

To continue on with irony, honey, even despite its taste being sweet, is one of the few sweeteners that the *kapha dosha* can consume regularly. I do, however, recommend moderation here. Honey is easy to digest since it is pre-digested by the bee and does have a warming post-digestive effect on the body. The *vata* type, and especially the *pitta* type should avoid or limit the consumption of honey - more so during the summer.

Kapha Sample Routine

Awaken: 5:00 a.m. YIKES!

Clean Teeth & Mouth: 5:15 a.m.

Consume Warm Water (w/ lemon): a few minutes following the cleaning of your teeth and mouth

Yoga or Meditation: 5:30 a.m.

Bathe & Self-Oil Treatment (*abhyanga*): 6:30 a.m.

Breakfast (1st meal of the day): 7:00 a.m. or skipping breakfast is okay

Lunch (2nd meal of the day): Noontime - 1:00 p.m.

Dinner (3rd meal of the day): 7:00 p.m. - 8:00 p.m.

Bedtime: 11:00 p.m. - sleep on your left side or back (barring injury)

The human body has the inherent ability to easily adapt and it loves routine and repetition. The *kapha* type welcomes routine more than the other three body-types, so slightly varying the times and routine for the above can have a balancing effect. This, of course, will be needed to be looked at on a specific case-by-case basis. Drastic deviations, however, can cause and or increase any imbalance, so slight and mild changes are always the safer way to introduce change into your daily routine.

Sample Kapha Meal Plan - Winter

Breakfast:

grapefruit sweetened with honey

seasonsoned with ginger and cardamom

or

hot cereal with ginger, honey and cinnamon

with

warm water & lemon or ginger, coriander and fennel tea

Lunch:

carrot soup seasoned with black pepper and ginger

or

chickpea with a coconut pesto

with

warm water or lemon or ginger, coriander and fennel tea

Dinner:

quinoa with garlic, ginger and red onion

or

spicy mung dal kitchari, with broccoli and cauliflower seasoned with cumin

with

ginger, coriander and fennel tea

Sample Exercise Routine - Kapha

Like the *kapha* pacifying diet, your exercise routine should be centered around movement and intensity. The *kapha* type possesses a great deal of dormant energy, thus allowing the ability to thrive during strenuous exercise. By activating this stored energy, you are, in fact, burning off the excess water and earth elements. By doing so, you are naturally fostering a healthy weight. By increasing both the duration and intensity of your workouts, you will more easily become accustomed to the proper training regimen. At all times listen to your body! Yes, you need to get up and get moving and increase your workouts, but never at the cost of risking an injury. Proceeding at a slower pace at first will be an intricate part of your custom routine. As the weeks progress, so will the duration, intensity and difficulty of your workouts. If your current level of fitness is extremely low or you are suffering from an injury, than yoga will be a welcomed and beneficial option. A few suitable yoga poses would consist of the following; sun salutation (*surya namaskar*), warrior I (*virabhadrasana I*), warrior II (*virabhadrasana II*), reverse warrior (*viparita virabhadrasana*), as well as forward bends, and backward bends. Postures that stimulate metabolism such as cobra (*Bhujangasana*), bow (*dhanurasana*), side plank (*vasisthasana*), spinal rolls, and leg lifts are also very appropriate[51].

---

[51] "The Channel of the Mind - Banyan Botanicals." https://www.banyanbotanicals.com/info/ayurvedic-living/living-ayurveda/health-guides/the-channel-of-the-mind/. Accessed 18 May. 2018.

In addition to resistance training and a customized yoga routine, team sports and outdoor family activities are a great way to get up, get out and get moving. The sturdier and stockier build of the *kapha* type will excel at sports such as football, but activities like rollerblading on a sunny day are most suitable for balancing the earth and water elements. If you have or develop a passion for weight-training, and I am willing to bet you will, it needs to be performed in a fashion that incorporates a system of opposites. Here is a sample routine:

Monday - Chest & Shoulders
Tuesday - 30 minutes of two different aerobic exercises; running and mountain climbing
Wednesday - Yoga with 15-20 minutes of light cardio prior to class
Thursday - Rest
Friday - Arms & Back
Saturday - Legs & Abs
Sunday - Rest (taking a yoga class on your off days are suitable if energy levels are high)

The bottom line for all the *doshas*, especially *kapha dosha*, is to get active and stay active. Get off the couch, turn off your electronic devices and let's go! Remember, you do not need to join a gym or strictly train at a health club or with a personal trainer to stay active and fit. Simple pleasures such as walking is something that all of us need to start doing more throughout the day. Let us start today - lace up your sneakers, leave your doubts and excuses at the door, feel the warmth of the sun as it splashes on your face and let's go for a walk. I will see you outside!

The *vata dosha* will need to focus on maintaining a steady and predictable routine, but the more grounded nature of *Mr. & Mrs. Kapha Dosha*, must learn how to be delightfully unpredictable at times. As in all of the *tridoshas*, geographic area and climatic conditions are something that needs to be considered and respected. The cold and cooler nature of water and earth can benefit from a warmer and drier climate. Areas such as Riverdale, CA and San Diego, CA are just a few suitable geographic locations. Phoenix for some specific individuals would also be a wise choice. Given the intense heat of the summer months in Phoenix, AZ, even the cooler-natured *kapha dosha* needs to use caution and hydrate frequently - common sense prevails.

If you find yourself needing to reside in an unsuited area for your particular *dosha*, do not fear. By adopting an unyielding attitude towards the 3 Pillars of health, you will provide adequate aspects in order to balance certain climatic conditions in which you have little to no control of correcting. By focusing on specific times of your day, such as the early morning hours and consuming a larger lunch, will go further than you could've ever imagined for creating peace, harmony and balance. These positive changes are easy and can be intertwined throughout the hours of your days moving forward. Sure, most of us have developed bad habits throughout our years. Just as in the development of these bad habits we can, however, foster good habits moving forward. They're created in a similar manner as bad habits. You can unlearn and relearn in exactly the same fashion. During the creation of your specific customized version we will look, address and develop the specific intricacies of your true nature and your current challenges and overall goals.

An Ancient Medicine for Modern Times

"Yogaadapi visham tikshmuttam bheshajam bhavet,
bheshjam chaapi duryuktam tiksham sampadhyate visham"

Even an acute poison can become an excellent drug if it is properly administered.
On the other hand even a drug, if not properly administered,
becomes an acute poison.

योगादपिविषंतीक्ष्णमुत्तमं भेषजं भवेत्|
भेषजं चापि दुर्युक्तं तीक्ष्णं सम्पद्यते विषम्||१२६||

- **Charaka sutra sthana, Chapter 24, verse 126**

You are now aware of the concept and model of Ayurveda from a lifestyle point-of-view. In this chapter let's explore Ayurveda as a system of restoring health. Over the past few decades, our system of medicine here in the West has begun to adopt the principles of Ayurveda. Unbeknownst to most, as an example, most pharmaceutical pain relievers mimic and copy the natural properties of curcumin (the active ingredient in turmeric - curcuma longa). By focusing and by defining your goals only then can you begin to reveal the process of restoring balance to a state of dis-ease.

You want to be healthy, for a true state of health breeds happiness. If you find yourself desiring to be healthy, then we need to look at and define health, or better yet, wellness. I liken wellness to "an optimal balance of body, mind and spirit". One key factor to this definition is your understanding of what residing in a state of balance truly encompasses. We now understand and know that the term "balance" is purely subjective; for what is balancing for you can be aggravating for another, thus causing a state of imbalance. A state of health can be achieved through managing the ebb and flow of the energetic factors of nature. The aim of this system of health is that each individual must be responsible for managing and balancing these energetic patterns him or herself. This process develops and fosters an environment by which the laws of nature performs the healing - not a doctor or practitioner. Your responsibility is to recognize the cause and to effect the necessary change. How is this done? Simple...

Through the exploration of the certain distinct intricacies of the human body, we have created a system of medicine here in the West that breeds separateness. The West being a system of deductive medicine, whereas in the East they employ a philosophy of an inductive style. By maintaining a true state of health we need to focus on the universal, mental, physical, environmental and social aspects of life. You cannot...I repeat, you cannot affect change in one area without subsequently affecting change in other areas. A disruption to the equilibrium of any of these aspects will result in a state of disease or illness. Just as how water filling an ice cube tray spills from one area to the next, the longer a disruption is ignored, the further the disturbance will expand and grow making it difficult to return the system to a state of ease.

The evolution of modern technology has made it possible to treat physical damage, structural damage, and diseases that require extreme interventions effectively. Eastern traditions, however, bring forth the knowledge and skills on how to promote healing in the individual, as well as the community as a whole, through the timeless philosophies of holistic methodologies.

Concept of Change

The act of change is a threefold process, or I should say, should be viewed as a three step process. A systematic process of change exists on both the gross and subtle levels of nuure, of which the human body exists on the gross plane of manifestation. The three principles are as follows:

1. The factor that causes the change
2. The aspect that undergoes the change
3. The responsible principle that brings these two together and which controls and regulates the law of cause and effect

When looking to treat disease and restore balance the above must be recognized and understood. Each result is born out of the prior result. This concept dates back to the origins of life and of the universe itself. Just as everything in the universe is connected, all of your organs, tissues and bones are interconnected and work in unison and in harmony with the whole. You cannot singularly treat disease. Likewise, you cannot ingest a pharmaceutical for gout without affecting all areas and aspects of the body and the mind.

Taking a pill may in fact help subside certain physical manifestations, but it also, however, creates a disturbance within the energetic blueprint of the trinity. By treating disease in this fashion we effect change on the gross level, but create disturbances on the subtle level, which in turn will develop further changes within the gross level itself.

When looking at instituting change within the human body, Ayurveda has a very scientific and practical system. Change is broken down into 3 categories of therapy, all of which are centered around the vitiation of the *doshas* and their respective *subdoshas*. The 3 categories of treatment are spiritual, rational and psychological disorders. Spiritual therapy consists of the recitation of mantras, auspicious acts, offerings & gifts, following religious precepts, atonement, fasting and invoking blessings. The rational model of therapy, however, is centered around the incorporation of herbs and other organic medicines, as well as the union of a diet and lifestyle centered around one's unique constitution and its current state of health (*vikruti*). Finally, psychological therapies are based on the restraint of the unwholesome objects of the mind and replacing them with wholesome objects. An object in this context can be best likened to our thoughts. Ask yourself, what is the opposite of anger, hate and resentment? Replace those unwhole objects with objects of an opposite nature - the Universe will take care of the rest!

The Treatment Process

The qualities and aspects of the treatment should be the opposite nature of the imbalance. The methods contained above are simple and straightforward; you treat cold with hot, dry with wet or gooey and dull with sharp. The types of medicines within this framework are looked upon as medicines that increase or decrease the vitiated *dosha* and medicines that maintain its state of homeostasis. It is important to note here, however, that medicines can also aggravate and cause a *doshic* disturbance. Just because it is "medicine" does not mean that is will always promote health and never cause disease. Actually, the contrary is more common than not, just listen to the end of any pharmaceutical advertisement.

Since the aspects of qualities in general are critical to our health, looking at the qualities of the medicinal formulations should be no different. The 3 categories of medicinal substances according to Ayurveda are substances of animal origin, plant origin and mineral origin.

1. **Animal Origin** - medicines from an animal origin will consist of substances such as honey, bone, muscle, dairy, fats, bile, skin, semen, horn and nail, just to list a few

2. **Plant Origin** - medicines from plant origin will consist of the flower, leaf, stem, and root

3. **Mineral Origin** - medicines from a mineral origin will consist of gold, silver, copper, iron, lead, silica, salt. Any substance obtained from under the earth as well as their by-products can be classified as a substance from a mineral-based origin. Even substances which are known to be dangerous, like arsenic, can be used medicinally if properly prepared.*

The goal of any treatment, as it was so formally established within concepts of Ayurveda, is the process of restoring balance to the *doshas*. One important aspect to the maintenance and balancing of the *doshas* is the proper management of the disorder itself. The executives of therapy should be employed as a means of balancing the mind and body via a systematic process of treatment. The management of any disorder is threefold; (1) the extraction (2) purification (3) avoidance of all etiological factors. The utilization of this form of therapeutic management will able you to successfully remove any toxins or by-products of the illness, purify the body and its various organs and tissues, as well as ensure the imbalance does not reoccur by engaging in the same or similar behaviors which first caused an aggravation of the *doshas*. By looking upon treatment that encompasses a system of opposites, the body then automatically begins to restore itself to a process of homeostasis. This happens automatically, without any thought or effort on your part - this is the beauty of Ayurveda and life itself.

*Note, I am not recommending the administering of any "medicinal" substances without the guidance of a licensed physician or certified practitioner.

Detoxification

The human body is a highly intelligent and very hard working organism but even despite its brilliance, it does get overtaxed. When the natural biological functions of the human body become impaired or when we begin to experience a vitiation of any of the *doshas*, build up of various toxins and by-products will follow. So it stands to reason that the first step in the treatment of any disorder is the removal of toxins that have accumulated during the aggravation of the *doshas*. When looking to accomplish the first step of the treatment process, you need to be aware that there are two separate aspects which need to be considered; internal and external aspects of the whole. Internal therapies can be best likened to any modality which purges the internal tissues, blood and organs of the body. The consumption of herbs with expectorant and diuretic properties, raw juices, vomiting and enemas are all ways to help purge the interior of the body from toxic accumulation and *ama*. External purging can include actions like massage or pressing actions, fomentation, sprinkling and pasting of various medicinal formulas. The specific action, of course, even down to the oil used in massage therapy, needs to be specific to your *dosha* and its current state (*vikruti*). There are certain characteristics and procedures that can be likened to both an internal and an external therapies that can be utilized if and when needed. Actions such as applying leeches to the skin was used often in ancient times as a way to cleanse the blood. Blood letting was also widely used during this particular period, however, it is rarely used today and this author does not recommend it as the safest option for purifying the blood.

Benefits of Cleansing

It is no secret that detoxing and cleansing is not only beneficial for the body and mind, but it is also a must. Whether the procedure is an ancient Ayurvedic tradition, a modern modality or a naturally occurring function of the human body, the clearing of our tissues, organs, channels and mind is something that should be performed regularly. Just as in the disease process itself, the longer the buildup of toxins is allowed to accumulate within the body and mind, the more comprehensive the treatment will need to be in order to address the imbalance. The practice of cleansing is considered a vital part of any lifestyle with great potential for improved energy, strength, immunity, as well as a renewed love of life. Here is a brief breakdown of the benefits of detoxification via an Ayurvedic perspective:

- Restores a sense of calm to the mind and the nervous system
- Nurtures an improved sense of energy, vitality and enthusiasm for life
- Supports the maintenance of a healthy body weight
- Helps to restore and maintain balanced sleep cycles
- Promotes regular and balanced elimination
- Helps to recover each individual's natural state of balance
- Prepares the tissues for deep nourishment and rejuvenation
- Promotes optimal health
- Fosters both clarity and groundedness in the mental, spiritual and emotional spheres. The therapeutic aim of a cleanse within the framework of Ayurveda is to pull toxins from the tissue and organs and into the digestive tract in order to be successfully carried out of

the body. The process of such can sometimes cause unpleasantness. Often times the detoxification procedure itself is taken as a manifestation of an illness due to the fact that the impurities can become palatable. This is short lived and once it passes the positive benefits from the cleanse can begin to be experienced.

There are 4 distinct phases of a cleanse mentioned within the scope of Ayurveda. The four phases are as follows:

1. **Preparation** - This first step of the detox process is important in order to prepare your body as well as your mind for the ensuing cleanse. This is achieved by choosing the optimal time based upon your specific schedule, your specific *dosha* and the time of year. In addition, ensuring you are mentally prepared is also critical to the success of the detox. It is important to note here that menstruating women want to plan their cleanse around their cycle. It is possible to activate your menstrual cycle during a cleanse. If this were to happen, suspend all cleanse activities except the dietary guidelines. The addition of self-massage during this part of your cleanse is advised. This is referred to as *abhyanga* in Ayurveda.

2. **Active Cleansing** - This is the heart of the process. During this stage you'll consume only foods that constitute higher detoxification properties, that are *dosha* specific, easy to digest and nourishing. This is normally accompanied by a slight caloric reduction and a slight

increase of water or raw juice, but certainly not always and not for everyone. This stage is designed to give our often overworked digestive system time to catch up and begin to restore itself to optimal working capacity. The addition of *triphala* (translates to the 3 flowers; *almalaki, harataki & bibalaki*) into your diet is advised. I recommend doing so in the form of tea.

3. **Reintroduction** - This ever crucial step is where you are to slowly wean yourself back onto your *dosha* specific diet. The slow reintroduction of harder to digest foods are consumed. It is important during this phase to slowly incorporate foods with a high allergen potential such as nuts and foods containing wheat. The methodical reintroduction of certain foods revs up your digestive fire, thus making sure it is functioning optimally moving forward.

4. **Purification** - During this final phase of your cleanse, you'll focus on the nourishment of plasma, blood, bone and other tissues in order to ensure the reproduction of new cell growth. This promotes stability and rejuvenation of systems and organs which had become impaired prior to the cleanse.

During the customized version of this work I will include the specific steps which will be created around you and your challenges, *dosha* and goals. This will include a detailed step-by-step process, specific recipes, as well as access to email consultations. Like any health-related modality, the individualized nature must be brought forefront in order to ensure your success and safety - cleanses and detoxes are surely no exception to this rule.

Diet & Cleansing

One of the best forms on an internal therapy I could ever recommend is ironically the least comprehensive, easiest and least expensive option available to man. You may be wondering at this point what that could be? It is simple, diet! The simple addition or subtraction of certain foods has not only cleansing and purification properties, but also nourishes and supports life simultaneously. Imagine how wonderful it would be if the gas or fuel added to your car also cleaned the interior and exterior of your vehicle at the same time? Mr. Sparkle, I'm sure, would not be happy!

The main goal of consuming any food should be the nourishment and detoxification of the body and mind. When looking at diets there have been many which have been successful in various areas and for various reasons. Diets like the Keto Diet and Atkins Diet have documented success, especially in the areas of weight-loss and reduction. Should the only goal of diet be merely dropping a few pounds? The obvious answer to that is no! When looking at these common diets none have successfully proven long-term stability in growth, nourishment and detoxification. Finding successful ways of promoting long-term maintenance is important if dietary interventions are going to have a significant health benefit. This is where the model of Ayurveda can prove to be an extremely beneficial system of promoting longevity and health, of which weight-loss is a positive by-product.

There are countless and well documented foods and herbs that have extremely high detoxification properties. *Ashwagandha* is an herb with extremely high detoxification properties. There is one herb in particular, which although very well known and widely used in Ayurvedic circles, is also well known and used in our culture and in various South American cultures. This is an herb which becomes important to consume regularly if you eat a lot of fish, especially fish which is known to contain higher traces of mercury. Cilantro has been used for many generations as a detoxifying agent. Fish is not the only exposure to mercury we come in contact with regularly. If you've had a cavity filled around the 1980's then you're exposed to mercury everyday of your life. Mercury can also be found in pharmaceutical medications, our water supply, manufactured products and even in air pollution. When heavy metals accumulate to reach toxic levels, they can lead to an array of symptoms and chronic conditions. The chemical compounds in cilantro act as natural cleansing agents, binding to toxic metals and loosening them for easy transport out of the body.

Another great herb possessing high detoxifying properties is also well known, however, it is not best known as an herb but rather a weed. Look outside during the summer and unless you spend a decent amount of money on landscaping, it is more times than not growing effortlessly in your backyard. Dandelion has traditionally been used as a diuretic and preliminary research suggests that it may help improve liver and gallbladder function. Of noteworthy nutritional value, dandelion is chock full of vitamins A, B6, C, D and K plus minerals, such as iron, potassium, zinc, and higher levels of beta carotene than carrots[52]. Dandelion is truly a wonder, in that all parts of the plant, including the root and stem can be used medicinally and are safe to consume. You will learn more about this super-weed in Part II of this work.

Another common and very well documented herb that possesses great detoxification properties is turmeric. I could write an entire volume on the medicinal value and uses of turmeric, and I am sure this has already been done. Among the over 500 medicinal values of curcumin, one of the least known is its detoxification value. Turmeric stimulates the gallbladder to produce bile. Bile, if you aren't already aware, eliminates toxins in the liver and rejuvenates cells that break down harmful compounds. Couple this with its very well documented anti-inflammatory properties and you cannot go wrong by adding this wonder root into your diet. Of course, over consumption, like anything, can create an imbalance. Oh, and turmeric is fat soluble, not water soluble - so take with healthy fats!

One last herb, actually it is an herbal formula, that I would like to mention here, is *triphala*. This wonderful polyherbal preparation is one of the most effective detox formulas ever made. It has been used successfully for centuries under the umbrella of Ayurveda, not to mention its ever increasing popularity

---

[52] Collins JM and Miller DR. Dandelion green bezoar following antrectomy and vagotomy - case report. J Kansas Med Soc 1966;67(6):303-304.

here in North America. It consists of three separate fruits, as mentioned earlier. Its efficacy stems around its digestive and cleaning action, especially to the bowels. What makes this preparation so effective is the fact that it is *tridoshic*, meaning under proper use and application it is balancing for the *doshas*. The unique combination of *amalaki, haritaki* and *bibhitaki* is a potent formula that has amazing anti-inflammatory properties, as well as being touted for being antiviral and antibacterial. Given these qualities and the tonic energetics, *triphala* can be considered for use in the very young, the infirmed and the elderly. Other classical Ayurvedic classifications attributed to the formula are the fact that it is also a digestive, mild laxative (normal doses), bowel tonic (low dose), purgative (high doses), carminative, expectorant, antispasmodic and bronchodilator. In addition, there are a myriad of other uses that are described, both in the Ayurvedic medical literature and anecdotally[53].

Panchakarma - the 5 Actions

When *ama* accumulates within the body it blocks the channels where the movement of energy, information and nutrients flow throughout the system. This is one of the main reasons why maintaining an optimal digestive state is so critical to your overall health. When this process breaks down, however, cleansing and purging the body of *ama* and other impurities becomes imperative. As you've already learned, Ayurveda links this to the cause of all disease.

---

[53] "Therapeutic Uses of Triphala in Ayurvedic Medicine - NCBI." 1 Aug. 2017, https://www.ncbi.nlm.nih.gov/pmc/articles/PMC5567597/. Accessed 20 May. 2018.

When looking at detoxification as a therapeutic action, Ayurveda fosters one of the more effective detox procedures called *panchakarma*. *Panchakarma* loosely translated in English means "5 actions". There are five purification procedures which make up this popular form of therapy. Here in the US, *panchakarma*, other than perhaps yoga, is the most widely known aspect of this ancient form of medicine. Foster a robust mental and physical digestion and experience good health. When you find yourself suffering from an impaired digestive state, *panchakarma* then becomes the first step in the correction of the imbalance and removal of *ama* and other various accumulated toxins. This timeless therapy of Ayurveda can help by reversing the negative effects of daily life. It can restore your natural state of health and wellness by cleansing your body of toxins, bringing balance into your system and improving bodily function.

The name, "5 steps" can be somewhat misleading given the fact that I recommend 2 intial steps which are used to prepare the body for the process itself. Before making any changes to your system or preparing to introduce or reintroduce any foods or medicines, the body needs a short period of preparation and adjustment. You can liken this to walking into the gym and warming up and stretching (in that order, please) before starting your routine. The first 2 warmup steps will consist of *snehan* and *svedana*. *Snehan* is a medicated oil massage that is effective in the moving of toxins into the gastrointestinal tract, as well as softening the superficial layers of the epidermis. This process helps reduce stress and relaxes the nervous system. I recommend performing this for 2-3 days prior to the start of the treatment.

On the last day of *snehan* you will want to perform *svedana*, or in everyday terms, sweat it out, baby! Through the process of sudation toxins are further liquefied which increases the movement of toxins into the gastrointestinal tract. Once this has been successfully performed, you should immediately begin the process of *panchakarma* to ensure that there is no further build up of toxins. Here are the five steps of *panchakarma*:

1. **Basti** = Herbalized Oil Enemas
2. **Nasya** = Nasal Irrigation
3. **Vamana** = Therapeutic Vomiting
4. **Virechana** = Purgation
5. **Raktamokshana** = Bloodletting

Yes, I know a few of the above procedures do not sound pleasant, and as I've already mentioned earlier in this chapter, bloodletting is not recommended by this author. If this procedure is a must than it needs to be performed by a licensed physician or practitioner - no exceptions here! I am going to take a few moments to break down the above procedures in order to help further your understanding of why these steps are necessary, as well as to educate you as to their efficacy.

Basti or Oil-based Enema: The colon is the main site in the body where the *vata dosha* resides, and since the *vata dosha* can oftentimes be the active principle in the pathogenesis of disease, this step becomes a critical action in the removal of toxins and for balancing of the *vata dosha*. Vata is the main etiological factor in the manifestation of disease since it is the "movement" endeavor within the body. *Vata* is mainly located in the large intestine, but bone tissue (*asthi dhatu*) is also a sub-seat of this *dosha*. Hence the medication administered rectally effects *asthi dhatu*. The mucus membrane of the colon is related to the outer covering of the bones (periosteum), which nourishes the bones. Any medication, therefore, given rectally is absorbed more easily and effectively. The herbal formulas being administered during this step must be suited to your specific *dosha* and the imbalance. The formula for the *basti* you'll need to use will be provided in your customized version of this book if you should choose so.

Nasya or Nasal Irrigation: It has often been said that the nose is the gateway to the brain, and seeing as how sinus, throat and nose issues have become so prevalent today, administering specific medicines directly into the nasal passage becomes a very effective treatment and has been used for many generations as a form of detoxification. The life force *prana* enters the body via the food we consume, as well as through breaths taken in via the nose. From here it enters the brain where it governs certain mental and cognitive functions. The efficacy of *nasya* lies in the fact that it acts both at local and systemic levels. Recent trends in modern science are emphasizing the use of transnasal routes for the administration of drugs as the nasal mucosa constitute the only site in the body that provides a direct connection between central nervous system and the atmosphere[54]. Drugs administered to the nasal cavity rapidly transfer to the cribriform plate and then to the central nervous

---

[54] "Nasal route and drug delivery systems. - NCBI." https://www.ncbi.nlm.nih.gov/pubmed/15230360. Accessed 20 May. 2018.

system via three routes; directly via olfactory neurons, via supporting cells and the surrounding capillary bed, directly through cerebrospinal l fluid[55]. Ghee, or clarified butter is the most common carrier in the administration of medicinals into the nasal passages, but again, this also should be *dosha* specific.

Vamana or Therapeutic Vomiting: If you've ever found yourself suffering from excess mucus in your lungs, throat and nasal passages, this is a strong indicator of an excess of the *kapha* dosha. The go to treatment for thousands of years within the framework of Ayurveda to help reduce the accumulation of *kapha* has been vomiting. Yes, I know what you're thinking because I am also one who hates to vomit. We must ask ourselves if a few brief moments of unpleasantness is worth relieving days upon days of feeling sick? *Kapha* disorders and associated *pitta* disorders originating or settled in the seats of these two respective *doshas* will be relieved either permanently or for long periods of time. Vomiting helps to prevent the forthcoming of disorders due to the vitiation *kapha* and *pitta*. Most Ayurvedic drugs are administered orally. First it goes to the stomach (*amashaya*), which is the main seat of *kapha* in the body. The digestion of food starts in the stomach. If there is an accumulation or aggravation of *kapha* in the stomach, the digestion of foods or drugs does not properly take place. With the help of *vamana karma*, a

---

[55] Sangeeta HJ, Toshikhane HD. A critical evaluation of the concept of "Nasa Hi Shiraso Dwaram" (Nasal Route Entry for the Cranial Cavity) Pac J Sci Technol. 2009;10:338–41.

deeper cleansing occurs, so the digestion of drugs and food happens successfully[56].

Virechana or Purgation: When excess bile is present in the liver, gallbladder and small intestine it is an indication of a vitiation of the *pitta dosha*. Excess bile can lead to manifestations such as jaundice, rashes, inflammation of the skin, as well as vomiting and fever. It clearly states in the Ayurvedic literature that when these physical manifestations are present the administration, purgation or a therapeutic laxative is to be used. Purgatives help reduce the excess *pitta* causing a decrease of bile. Purgatives can, in fact, completely relieve the excess accumulation of *pitta*. When using purgatives you should avoid foods that will aggravate the predominant humor or cause the three humors to become unbalanced. This is the case when performing any of the 5 actions of *panchakarma*.

Raktamokshana or Bloodletting: Toxemia is a common condition where the toxic byproducts from the GI tract enter the bloodstream. This can often be the cause of chronic infections as well as hypertension and other circulatory disorders. Eczema is not only a common issue relating directly to an imbalance of the blood, but is also a disorder which hosts many psychologically related issues. Not only are skin disorders embarrassing for the many who suffer from them, but they're typically painful due to the fact that the skin is a very sensitive organ. *Pitta* is produced from the disintegrated red

---

[56] "A study on Vasantika Vamana (therapeutic emesis in ... - NCBI." https://www.ncbi.nlm.nih.gov/pmc/articles/PMC3296337/. Accessed 21 May. 2018.

blood cells in the liver. So *pitta's* relationship to blood is very close. An accumulation of *pitta* can build up into the blood causing toxicity, and thus many *pitta* disorders. Extracting a small amount of blood from a vein relieves the tension created by the increased toxins in the blood. I mentioned before that I am not a fan of this step, however, certain cases may require this sensitive procedure. If the manifestation is minor, this author would suggest blood-leeching. Leeches have been used as an alternative to bloodletting in both ancient traditions as well as in modern applications of *panchakarma*. Bloodletting or leeching also stimulates the spleen to produce anti-toxic substances that help to stimulate the immune system. Toxins are neutralized enabling radical cures in many blood-borne disorders[57].

The duration of your cleanse is another important aspect that needs to be *doshic* and individual specific. There are various other factors that will need to be considered here such as lifestyle, especially your work and leisure routines. This is an aspect that will be created and documented during your customized version of this book, however, 3-5 days are best. This generalization does not include the 2 pre-cleanse steps mentioned earlier in this chapter. You will need to be in greater communication with your body during any period of cleansing. Doing will will advise you when to begin, when to stop and when to continue. These important consideration will help shape and form the specific duration of your detox. It is also not uncommon for your subsequent cleanses to be shorter and more successful than your first performance. Like

---

[57] Aacharya Vaidya Jadavaji Trikamji., editor. Vol. 24. Varanasi: Chaukhamba Sanskrit Sansthan; 1990. Charaka, Charakasamhita, Sutrasthana, Vidhishonitiya Adhyaya; p.12

anything, the more we as humans do, the more we do it the better and easier it becomes. You've got to love the brilliance of neuroplasticity!

One important aspect of any cleanse is proper rest. The removal of toxins does require proper rest and proper nutrition. Typically during any cleansing process you'll experience lower levels of energy. This is your body's way of letting you know to take it easy and relax as often as possible. I do not advise any exercise, especially heavy resistance training or high impact movements during your detox. Walking and certain forms of yoga can be advantageous during your detox if you feel the need to exercise. Excessive exposure to stimulus like loud music or television also should be reduced or avoided. Remember, we need to mentally digest any and all bits of information coming into the body via the five senses. Just take a few moments to remind yourself of the goal of your cleanse - once this endeavor floats forefront into your mind, you should be able to successfully navigate the waters of your cleansing periods successfully and effortlessly.

Panchakarma is a delicate process which needs to be performed correctly and customized to meet the needs, challenges and of course, *dosha* of each individual. I would advise consulting with a seasoned Ayurvedic Practitioner with this process to ensure both your safety and success. Proper safety and the greater assurance of success - what could possibly create any greater of an outcome for your next detox?

Ayurveda Therapeutics

The preservation of the equilibrium of the *dhatus* not only promotes health, but helps fight against disease. The goal of treatment unbeknownst to most, but should be the foundation of your approach, is the elimination of the disequilibrium of the *doshas*. From this standpoint, medicinals and herbal remedies are to be looked upon in two ways; one that maintains health or corrects the abnormalities of the *dosha*. As mentioned prior, there are 3 forms of medicines within the scope of Ayurveda. In this section we will deal with medicines of plant origin.

When looking at the pharmacological efficacy of herbal remedies and formulas, one very important distinction that needs to be understood is the synergistic nature of these organic compounds. When consuming herbal compounds or even organic foods for that matter, a single herb may contain more than one phytochemical constituents, which works in harmony with each other in producing the specific pharmacological action[58]. This is precisely the reason why most Ayurvedic herbal preparations are produced via the combination of several herbal compounds. As an example, ginger can be best paired with black pepper and long pepper in order to increase its efficacy in treatment and the removal of excess mucus. Combining these three singular plant-based compounds increases the action of heat. The heating action of this particular formula offers an opposite effect which lead to the excess of phlegm and mucus; accumulation of the *kapha dosha*. Cumin, black

---

[58] Meena AK, Bansal P, Kumar S. Plants-herbal wealth as a potential source of ayurvedic drugs. Asian J Tradit Med. 2009;4:152–70.

pepper and asafoetida are used together traditionally to reduce bloating due to weak digestion; whereas guduchi and turmeric combinated boosts one's immunity[59].

The nature and specific action of the synergistic properties of any given herbal or bio-herbal based formula is divided into two separate categories: formulas working together to increase its rate of absorption, distribution, metabolism and elimination. The second category is based upon how the compounds of the formula are received by the various receptors of certain physiological systems[60]. As a reminder, just because you are consuming any given food or medicine certainly does not ensure that it will work in the manner in which it was intended. As an example, turmeric / curcumin is not water soluble, thus needs to be consumed with fats. I have seen so many people waste good money on taking curcumin supplements in the morning with water on an empty stomach and then they wonder why their feces turns rust-colored. Remember when I stated that for each meal you must invite the "Shuns" over? Well, this same principle holds true when consuming medicines, especially those of a plant, animal or mineral origin.

In *Ayurveda*, herbals are known to regulate bodily functions, cleanse and nourish the human body. Each herb has five categories known as their taste

---

[59] Pole S. London: Jessica Kingsley Publishers; 2013. Ayurvedic Medicine: The Principles of Traditional Practice

[60] Chorgade MS. Drug Discovery and Development. Vol. 2. Hoboken, New Jersey: John Wiley and Sons Inc; 2007. Drug development.

(*rasa*), the energy an herb releases when ingested (*veerya*), their post-digested effect (*vipaka*), special and unique power of an herb that has variable action (*prabhava*) and their therapeutic action (*karma*). The time of day the herbal medicine is taken, along with the specific dosage and the carrier used will need to be specific to you, your unique bodily humor and its current state of health. Ghee, water and honey, however, are a few of the more common carriers of medicinal formulas.

From this point, there are two distinct classifications of herbal formulas: pure herbal formulas and bio-herbal formulas, which are plant-based formulas with the addition of medicines from a mineral-based origin. The Sanskrit term for these two types are *kasthoushadhies* and *rasaushadhies* (herbal-bio-mineral metallic preparation), in which the latter contains minerals added for their therapeutic effect[61].

Just as in the compatibility of certain foods, the formulation of certain medicinal preparations can also become incompatible (*viruddha*) when consumed together, and thus should be avoided. The nature of the incompatibility can reside in either a quantitative incompatibility, energetic incompatibility or functional incompatibility. As an example, ghee should not be taken in the same proportions with honey by weight due to conflicting tastes and temperatures; laxatives and astringents when combined together

---

[61] Chaudhary A, Singh N. Herbo mineral formulations (rasaoushadhies) of ayurveda an amazing inheritance of ayurvedic pharmaceutics. Anc Sci Life. 2010;30:18–26.

create an antagonistic action in which they negate each other's activities[62]. The energetic action of the phytonutrients when combined with certain energetic qualities of other compounds affects the human body on an energetic and cellular level. In addition, most Ayurvedic formulas cause far less side effects and are typically safer for the environment. Not to mention, they're less expensive than their chemical counterparts. With this said, however, the careless combining and consumption of any medicine of any origin is not condoned by this author. Like any health-related procedure or intervention, always consult your doctor or certified practitioner when preparing to consume herbal-based medicines and formulas. This is especially important when dealing with formulas containing compounds such as heavy metals. One last important issue that you need to be aware of is the manufacturing practices of herbal formula, be it Ayurvedic-based or not. Purchasing products from a licensed manufacturer is a detail that needs to be addressed. This is not only true of our medicines, but our foods as well. Working with a certified or licensed physician in most cases will reduce the likelihood or consuming poorly prepared and manufactured formulas, as well as reduce the risk of cross contamination. Remember, always err on the side of caution when it comes to your health and well-being!

---

[62] Pole S. London: Jessica Kingsley Publishers; 2013. Ayurvedic Medicine: The Principles of Traditional Practice

Mental Therapies

When looking at treating any imbalance or malady there is more times than not that a mental or psychological aspect that needs to be addressed. The traditions of Ayurveda understands this better than any other form of healing. Even the term "*Ayus*" of which forms the root word "*Ayur*" means life, or it is said that "life" is the combined state of body, sense, mind and soul. Ayurveda has duly recognized the individuality of psyche (*manas*) and body (*sarera*) and their inseparable and interdependent relationship within a living organism. The importance of mind even outside the realm of a therapeutic model is mentioned and well documented throughout the ancient texts. For instance, the role of the mind (*manas*) in the digestion of food consumed is stressed. Ayurveda advises that food should be consumed with rapt attention, or as it is referred to today, mindfulness. When the proper attention is not placed upon the art of eating, digestive disturbances are sure to follow.

Indicating the need for the proper state of mental health for the efficacy of proper drug action Ayurveda states that "no one who has not rid oneself of the evils of both mind and body beginning with the gross ones, can ever expect to reap the benefits resulting from vitalization therapy"[63]. These straightforward statements are not only precise in their meaning, but are also a strong indication that this ancient system of medicine was the first to document the action of the mind in the treatment of both physiological and psychological disorders. The mind is a psycho-motor entity, in the fact that it

---

[63] Acharya, Y.T., "Charaka Samhita", Nirnayasagar Press. Bombay, 338. (1938)

possesses both action and quality, coexistent within itself. In Ayurveda this is referred to as *ubhayatmaka*[64].

When looking at disorders of the mind, just as in Ayurveda's approach to the physical body, disease stems from a derangement of the three mental *doshas* of the mind; *sattva, rajas,* and *tamas*. I have often been asked why the difference in the reference of the mental versus bodily humors. Manas has two basic qualities which are referred to in the ancient texts as their atomic nature (*anutva*) and their unitary nature (*ekatva*). Like the concept of "*dosha*" itself, it is difficult to understand these qualities directly and clearly. Therefore, the mind within the framework of Ayurveda, is related to its three operational qualities, which are *sattva, rajas,* and *tamas*[65]. To further your understanding of the concept of the three *gunas*, you can think of them in terms of their mental response patterns. For instance, *satwa* is understood by self-control, knowledge, its discriminative ability and power of exposition. *Rajas* can be understood by violence, despotic envy, authoritativeness and experiences of self- adoration. *Tamas* is understood by dullness, non-action and sleep.

One aspect of mind which I will briefly touch upon here but will not go into too much detail, is the location of the mind. Take a few moments and poll a few strangers as to the whereabouts of the "mind". I am willing to bet that the most common response you'll garner is that the mind is located in the brain. Perhaps this common misconception is your current belief. The mind, under

---

[64] Acharya, Y.T., "Charakasamhita", Nirnayasagar Press, Bombay, 288. (1941)

[65] Shukla, G.D., "Bhelasamhita", Chowkhambha vidya Bhavan, Varanasi, 157. (1959)

the scope of Ayurveda, and I am also a huge proponent of this theory, is that the mind is located throughout the entire body. Taking this a step towards our current understanding of quantum physics, the mind can be likened to a holographic net which encompasses the entire being. The one main difference I would like to mention here, is that Ayurveda states that "mind" does not reside within the nail ends and hair[66]. The seat of the mind within the body is believed to be between the head and the heart, the heart being referred to as the seat of *Atman* or the soul.

Diseases are classified in three ways: (1.) disorders of a physical nature; (2.) disorders of a mental nature, and (3.) disorders of a psychosomatic nature. From a holistic viewpoint, which of course is consistent within the scope of Ayurveda, these arbitrary demarcations are made only for the clinical advantages. I would like to note here that it is not possible to strictly categorise diseases as physical or mental. When an organism experiences an imbalance, whether the imbalance manifests as mental or physical symptoms, any disorder affects the living body which is a combination of the body, senses, mind and soul. Remember, any part of the whole cannot experience a positive or negative change, for even if one of the three is deranged, the remaining three are also affected. This is law!

With the above in mind, the order of treatment needs to be clear and distinct. Any imbalance within the mind needs to first be addressed. As I've already mentioned in both this book and in another of my works (Law of One Mind),

---

[66] Acharya, Y.T., "Charakasamhita", Nirnayasagar Press, Bombay, 716. (1941)

"mind" is a very subtle aspect and cannot be thought of in physical terms. This does, however, make clinical diagnosis disorders related to the mind very difficult, especially for the layperson. When symptoms of a mental nature can be experienced and or classified, as you learned in the chapter "Pathology & Disease," the disease process has already manifested into the 3rd stage or beyond. This is where the difficulty lies. You're probably wondering what can be done? Simple, a monitoring of your thoughts - the things that go through your mind can be used as a diagnostic tool. The state of your mind is reflected via its function and form. Ask yourself, what has been your current temperament? What psychomotor activity or mental conduct have you been exhibiting? These aspects of the mind are grosser in their sensory transactions, thus allowing you to diagnose a derangement of the mind earlier within the stages of the disease process.

Ayurveda has classified 3 forms of mental treatment:

1. Spiritual Therapy
2. Logical Therapy
3. Psycho Therapy

The above therapies can be accomplished via mantras, prayer, wearing of sacred gems, medicines of a plant, animal & mineral origin, diet and lifestyle. Purification measures, such as *panchakarma*, are to be utilized, especially when there is an accompanying derangement of the *doshas*.

Like any physical imbalance, prevention of mental imbalances becomes the goal. The above mentioned are applicable when an accumulation of the *doshas* and or *gunas* has already begun. The importance of prevention relating to the mind can be found easily within the classical texts, especially under daily routine, diet and prevention of disease. In order to be free from mental disorders Ayurveda prescribes that one should not allow oneself to become a victim of impulses like greed, grief, fear, anger, jealousy, impudence, vanity etc. Further, the texts declares that one who speaks truth, refrains from overindulgence in alcohol and meat, hurts none, avoids overstrain, fair spoken, always compassionate and given to wholesome eating, would enjoy the benefits of sound mental health[67]. To sum up this section and this chapter as a whole - one who goes within daily, one who reacts to his fellow humans and the world around him in a positive light and one who foregoes grief for joy will experience perennial happiness.

---

[67] Paradhkar, "Astangahridaya" ,Nirnayasagar Bombay, 34. (1939).

Part II

Customize ME! - Ayurvedic Beauty

True Beauty Lives Within Dinacharya

"Triya Upstambha iti- Aaharah, swapno, brahmacharya miti, aibhistribhiryuktiyuktairupstabdhamupastambhayai shariram balvarnopchayopachitamnuvartateyaavadayu sanskaraat samskaramhitanupsevamanasya ya ihaivopdekshyate"

Healthy habits pertaining to food, sleep, and celibacy leads to good complexion, growth and full health for the full span of one's life.

त्रय उपस्तम्भा इति- आहारः, स्वप्नो, ब्रह्मचर्यमिति;
एभिस्त्रिभिर्युक्तियुक्तैरुपस्तब्धमुपस्तम्भैः शरीरं
बलवर्णोपचयोपचितमनुवर्त्ततेयावदायुःसंस्कारात्
संस्कारमहितमनुपसेवमानस्य, य इहैवोपदेक्ष्यते॥३५॥

- **Charaka sutra sthana, Chapter 11, verse 35**

The process of self-alignment of the mind and body to match the natural rhythms of the Universe is not only the foundation upon which Ayurveda was built, but it's also the foundation you'll need to establish when looking at art of beautification. The secret to the health of your hair, skin, nails, your weight and your smile (amongst others, of course) is what you do and do not do on a daily basis. The process of this alignment is referred to as *dinacharya* in Ayurveda.

Your daily routines, whether it is centered around a "beauty regimen" or is more focused on your career, pastime and meals, is an integral aspect of being human. Most of us have grown accustomed to doing things a certain way. Some consider this behavior to be a form of stubbornness, but it is essential to human survival. Ayurveda, of course, takes a much deeper look into one's daily routine and stresses it far more than we do here in the West. When looking at your daily beauty routine, this process takes a slightly different perspective, however, the two philosophies have one common goal; to help you look healthier and be the best you that you can be. It is important to take a few moments to look at the differences in your approach to beauty from those of the ancient traditions of Ayurveda.

A Timeless Paradigm of Beauty

In a time where beauty is looked upon as a practice of an outward to inward modality, the need to bring forth the true essence of "beauty care" could not come at a better time. Not only are today's modern attempts at beautification performed in an incorrect manner, the standard for beauty is also grossly misrepresented. Take a look at the cover of most beauty magazines today and the standard of excellence in beauty has certainly been clearly defined. Beauty has become a modality that is centered around merely our outward look and appearances, when nothing could be further from the truth! Let's take a moment and turn the clocks back, allowing our minds to expand as we travel to a time when beauty was defined under holistic terms.

Ayurveda's take on beauty closely mirrors a holistic approach to health. It's practices fall under the scope of one's daily routine (*dinacharya*) and is centered around diet, exercise and sleep. In addition, Charka considered cosmetics to be under the scope of medicine, meaning they're one in the same. Ayurveda breaks down beautification into three separate pillars; outer beauty (*roopam*), inner beauty (*gunam*) and lasting beauty (*vayastyag*). Under this model you cannot only think in terms of cosmetics to define or achieve a state of beauty. Good health and good nutrition thus controls the outward manifestation of beauty and your physical appearance. The key here is to understand that when you are living within a state of balance according to your specific nature, the health of your hair, vitality of your nails and the glow of your skin becomes a positive by-product. Radiant skin and a clear complexion stems from proper nutrition, adequate rest, a robust state of digestion and the successful elimination of waste and toxins. There is an old saying which states "that when diet is good, medicine is of no need. When diet is wrong, medicine is of no use." I am a firm believer that we can take this proclamation a step further by adding, "When diet is good, cosmetics are of no need. When diet is wrong, cosmetics are no help." Cover-up and mask as you like, however, can true beauty only be defined in this manner?

I want to be clear here in saying that even despite my current viewpoint, I am not against, nor am I suggesting that you should not enhance your look and appearance. I feel highlighting and defining our natural aspects of beauty is a blessing. This is where I will stray slightly from the ancient texts and will offer tips and suggestions on how to safely enhance your natural look. One area of cosmetics I feel needs to be addressed is the education in regards to the ingredients being used in man of today's beauty products and supplements. And surprising to most, not only are the lesser expensive products being manufactured with unsafe ingredients and chemicals, but many of the top and more expensive brands are inundated with potentially unsafe additives as well.

Avoiding toxins, as discussed earlier, is virtually impossible today. Most of us are aware of toxins via the foods we consume, but take a moment and ask yourself how many of us are aware of or are even concerned about the safety of the cosmetic products used on a daily basis? The sad fact is that most of your beauty and health-related products contain thousands of chemicals, many of which are being absorbed directly into your bloodstream. Remember, when a chemical or toxin is consumed via our food, water and air, the body has filtration systems in order to protect us from the harmful exposure of these foreign agents. The skin, however, is quite different; your skin is the only line of defense for thwarting external toxins from entering the bloodstream. Once absorbed through your skin, the chemicals entering your bloodstream are then carried throughout the entire body. One of the main areas of concern here is that many of them are manufactured to be highly absorbable, so in essence, the products themselves are designed to move the toxic and often dangerous chemicals effortlessly into the body. These various chemicals, and I will not get into many of them here, are skin irritants at best and endocrine disruptors and carcinogens at worst. Here is a list of five beauty additives that you should avoid which this author considers to be dangerous:

1. Parabens
2. Synthetic Colors
3. Phthalates
4. Formaldehyde
5. Propylene glycol

Does limited exposure offer a health risk? In most cases, no, limited and controlled exposure to any of the above will not have immediate adverse health ramifications. Now, if you are elderly, pregnant or are already suffering from disease, I would avoid them all together. If you find it impossible to avoid any of the above or any of the other potentially dangerous additives, proper diet, exercise and detoxification becomes critical. There are only 4 ways for toxicity to safely leave the body: urine, feces, vomiting and sweating. *Panchakarma*, as discussed in the chapter entitled "[An Ancient Medicine for Modern Times](#)," is one of the best methods of detoxification. If this is not possible for you at this time, then consume an adequate amount of water daily, get into the gym…and sweat! Oh, and limit your exposure when and where possible.

By opening the door to this ancient science you are in turn fostering a life centered around your true beauty and are flowing in accordance with nature. Through the further cultivation of the *tridoshic* principles of Ayurveda, we can begin to look at enhancing your already God-given pulchritudinous (a big shout out here to Woody Boyd!). There are certain things that needs to be performed daily for everyone, however, based on your unique constitution, its current state of health, the time of year and your geographic locale, the specific nature of these daily habits needs to change accordingly. Below is a list of actions that you need to consider adding into your daily routine - the specific nature of each will be provided in your customized version of this book. Here is my list of daily beauty suggestions:

- Consume a diet of fresh, organic & nutritious foods
- Consume *dosha* specific foods
- Get the appropriate amount of rest and sleep
- Exercise and sweat regularly
- Consume the adequate amount of properly filtered water
- Keep your body fit with exercise, for example, yoga *asanas*
- Avoid stress, overexertion and exhaustion
- Diffuse the proper essential oils and various aromatherapy methods
- Daily – or as often as possible – self-massage (*abhyanga*) with *dosha* specific oils
- Meditate as often as you can - this reduces stress in turn positively affecting your skin
- Decrease or eliminate chemical-based toiletries and various healthcare products by switching to organic-based cosmetics that are *dosha* specific

Skin Care

The desire to look beautiful is as old as the human race itself and the ancient literature of Ayurveda supports this proclamation. The use of certain plants and minerals are mentioned consistently throughout the treatises relating to beautification. There are numerous studies suggesting that even primitive cultures practiced the art of self-beautification[68]. The traditions of Ayurveda depended mainly upon plant and mineral-based cosmetics. There is the concept of *solah shringar*, meaning the "16 modes of beauty," in which a single or herbal composites are applied and used topically for the purpose of enhancing one's beauty. Herbs such as amla (emblica officinalis), turmeric (curcuma longa) and mango ginger (curcuma amada) have been used for centuries for their positive effects of beauty enhancement. For instance, the dry rhizome powder of the mango ginger root is used in facepacks in order to treat acne and other skin blemishes. Amla is a very popular Ayurvedic herb that has many medicinal uses. It is well known for balancing *pitta* and *kapha doshas* due to its sour and astringent energetics. It has been well documented as an effective diuretic, which is vital in the removal of toxins. Amla is also an excellent laxative. Under the scope of beautification, amla has been used for centuries as a hair and scalp tonic. Its powder can be used as a shampoo, whereas it has a scrubbing effect.

The important aspect to understand when looking at the efficacy of most cosmetics, is that the active compounds being used today are manufactured to

---

[68] "A History of Cosmetics from Ancient Times - Cosmeticsinfo.org." https://cosmeticsinfo.org/Ancient-history-cosmetics. Accessed 24 May. 2018.

mimic its naturally occurring counterpart. Why? Simple, it is far less expensive to manufacture synthetic compounds than it is to grow and harvest them naturally. In addition, no entity is allowed to copyright a naturally occurring compound. For many decades, manufacturers would then break down the active compounds, slightly changing its molecular structure, and voila - they have a unit that can be easily reproduced and trademarked. Well, according to the Supreme Court's decision in Association for *Molecular Pathology* v. *Myriad Genetics*, case 569 U.S on March 4th of 2013, this is now no longer allowed[69]. In my opinion, this is a huge step in not only the protection of the end user, but a step towards the majority of us looking to the timeless traditions of yesterday for our overall health, beauty and longevity. Okay, enough of the boring legal mumbo jumbo - let's move on.

Since most plant-based cosmetics are broken down into powders or tinctures, if they're to be successfully used topically they need to be used in conjunction with what is referred to as a carrier or base. Sesame oil is a common carrier often used in Ayurvedic traditions. Sesame oil contains two compounds called sesamin and sesamolin. They are biologically active and exhibit great oxidative properties[70]. In this light, sesame oil is used as an antioxidant and offers a moisturizing effect. One of my go-to carriers for topical use is ghee, more so ghee that has been washed 100 times. If you are unfamiliar with ghee that has been washed 100X, I recommend Googling it - it is marvelous! Facial masks

---

[69] "The New Patent Policy on Natural Products Is a Game ...." 16 Sep. 2014, https://www.bradley.com/insights/publications/2014/09/the-new-patent-policy-on-natural-products-is-a-g. Accessed 2 June. 2018.

[70] "Science Backs Ayurvedic Massage with Sesame Oil | John ...." 8 Oct. 2016, https://lifespa.com/science-backs-ayurvedic-massage-sesame-oil/. Accessed 2 June. 2018.

consisting of buttermilk or goat's milk are also excellent for skin applications. They both contain high amounts of vitamin A, B6, B12 and E, which are much safer and effective choices than chemically laden emollients. Saponin, which is a plant-based derivative, is also an excellent additive to any naturally occurring cosmetics. Any of these organic compounds should be used in place of petroleum and plastic derivatives. Significant evidence exists documenting the efficacy of plant and mineral-based skin care products for the treatment of psoriasis, eczema and acne vulgaris[71]. And of course, there is aloe vera that has been commonly used here in our culture after a long day at the beach. There is one common issue with aloe vera found here in the U.S - it is nowhere near pure aloe vera gel. In an article printed in the Chicago Tribune on the 11th of November, 2016 stated the following:

"Samples of store-brand aloe gel purchased at national retailers Wal-Mart, Target and CVS showed no indication of the plant in various lab tests. The products all listed aloe barbadensis leaf juice - another name for aloe vera - as either the No. 1 ingredient or No. 2 after water. There's no watchdog assuring that aloe products are what they say they are. The U.S. Food and Drug Administration doesn't approve cosmetics before they're sold and has never levied a fine for selling fake aloe."[72]

---

[71] Kapoor VP, Herbal cosmetics for skin and hair care, Natural product radiance, vol- 4 July-Aug 2007, 307-14

[72] "No evidence of aloe vera found in the aloe vera at Wal-Mart ...." 22 Nov. 2016, https://www.chicagotribune.com/business/ct-no-aloe-vera-lotion-wal-mart-cvs-target-20161122-story.html. Accessed 5 June. 2018.

Disturbing, to say the least - unsafe at the worst. Aloe vera is not the only plant-based herb used in relationship to the sun and sun bathing. Moringa oleifera, or as it is often referred to as the "drumstick tree" and "golden rain tree," has been used for centuries for its wide range of medicinal applications. Moringa is an excellent source of the essential amino acids as well as being very high in Vit. A. Moringa is a true wonder given that fact that it is antibacterial, antifungal and antiviral, thus making it a safer and effective alternative for protecting your skin from various infections. In recent clinical trials, products containing moringa oleifera blocked over 50% more harmful UV rays in relation to products containing no moringa whatsoever[73]. It's anti-proliferative effects were also tested and it demonstrated very positive results. Take a moment and ask yourself, would you rather lather your scalp and skin with products derived from petroleum or plastic, or would you prefer to use products containing this highly effective and safe herb which is sourced from Mother Nature?

The appearance, tonality and overall health of your skin is used in Ayurveda as a representation of the health and energetics of what is going on inside - more so, what is happening inside will be reflected on the outside. I have joked for years that if your skin is in rough shape I would hate to see what your liver looks like! By assessing the health of your skin and what skin-type you wear can offer clues as to whether or not you may be suffering from a derangement of the *tridoshas*. Knowing your skin-type affords you the chance to properly

---

[73] Fahey J.W. *Moringa oleifera*: A Review of the Medical Evidence for Its Nutritional, Therapeutic, and Prophylactic Properties. Part 1. Trees Life J. 2005;2005:1–5.

treat, nourish and diagnose common disorders. Here are the three skin types according to Ayurveda:

Vata Skin-Type - Those with this type of skin often experience their skin as being sensitive with a tendency to be paler and more susceptible to dryness than most other types of skin. The *vata* skin is typically thinner, thus making it prone to premature aging if not properly cared for and kept in a state of balance. Even despite this, it's far less prone to acne than the other two skin-types. Proper protection, hydration and nourishment are three essentials when looking at managing and treating this skin-type.

Pitta Skin-Type - If you hate the feeling of heat upon your skin than you most likely possess the skin of the *pitta*. The fiery nature of the *pitta dosha* makes this type of skin prone to sunburn and other various inflammatory related disorders like redness and acne. As I mentioned before, cool it down, especially in the warmer months of the year. The appearance of this skin-type type fosters a fairness with reddish undertones. It is more prone to acne than its *vata* counterpart and is known to emit a glowing quality when healthy. A diet consisting of a cooling nature in addition to oils and herbal formulas of the like are the means of treating and managing the fiery nature of this skin-type.

Kapha Skin-Type - The characteristics of this type of skin are unmistakable, being that this type of skin is fuller and thicker than the other two types. Having a tendency towards excessive oiliness and being cool and moist to the touch, means keeping these aspects of your skin in balance is a daily task that should not be overlooked. Having skin that is thick certainly helps fight off the signs of aging, however, because of its oily nature the *kapha* skin is prone to imbalances like cystic-acne. Daily cleansing with *kapha*-specific cleansers is a chore you need to perform daily. If not, the clogging of the pores can result in various skin eruptions, breakouts and fungal infections.

The proper management of stress, as it relates wholly to your entire physical, energetic and mental well-being, needs to be understood as it plays a vital role in the health of your skin. Those of us, like myself, who are predominantly of a fiery nature needs to be more disciplined than most in controlling and managing stress. When chronic stress is not properly managed it can cause an imbalance of the *doshas* (most often the *vata dosha*, but not always), thus manifesting at some point as a derangement of the skin. Some of the more common manifestations can be experienced as premature wrinkling of the skin and noticeable pigment changes. When you're residing in an emotional state of stress, the release of stress hormones is unavoidable. By continuing to live in a stressful state, the hormones of stress cause many disturbances of the body, thus manifesting as imperfections of the skin. Hormonal changes have been attributed to premature aging of the skin, excessive hair loss, acne, thinning of the skin, excessive sweating and diseases such as psoriasis and hives. Your skin is the parchment through which the language of your hormones is written upon. Ignore these physical signs and suffer from disease - read clearly the language of your skin and experience vibrant and healthy skin.

Skin Care, the Inside Out Approach

The appearance and health of your skin stems from your diet and lifestyle. When looking to manage and treat your skin, what goes in is what comes out. Lifestyle practices like going to bed on time and the quality of your sleep are factors that contribute to what you witness in the mirror each and every day. When looking at the inner to outer aspects of skin care this needs to be performed in accordance with your unique constitution and its current state (are you sick of hearing this yet...? Good, it is simply that important!). Like the health of your other various organs and tissues, Ayurveda has brought forth many excellent single and herbal compounds which have been used for thousands of years in the maintenance and treatment of the skin. Here are a few of the more common singular compounds and formulas:

Dandelion - Yes, that weed that grows in your yard each and every year without you having to do a damn thing. Dandelion supports the health of your digestive system, especially liver health, and thus is one of the best herbs when looking to treat and maintain the health of your skin. Dandelion is an excellent purifier of the blood and has wonderful detoxification properties. Dandelion is bitter in its taste and hosts a post digestive effective of a cooling nature, so it is excellent in taming the fiery nature of *pitta*-related disorders.

Burdock - Being another great herb in the detoxification of the liver, this wonder herb is a go to when looking to support the health of your skin. Burdock is one of the best "inside / out" options when looking towards the care and treatment of your skin. It works on treating the root cause of the internal aspects relating to the disruption of the *dosha* directly, thus making it great in the alleviation of skin disorders such as dandruff and eczema. Burdock is sweet and bitter, thus making it pacifying for *kapha* and *pitta*. It can be aggravating for *vata* due to that fact that it's qualities are dry and mobile.

Comfrey - Comfrey has a unique affinity for the health of your skin. It is easy to grow and is a very low maintenance herb that every garden should welcome with open arms. It is especially effective in the treatment of skin wounds, and is often found in first-aid kits in some form or another. Comfrey is rich in a compound called allantoin, which is what makes it an excellent choice in wound care, hence, giving it the nickname of "wound wart". The leaves of comfrey are astringent in taste, while its leaves are slightly sweeter making it possibly aggravating for *vata* and *kapha*. This is excellent for pacifying *pitta*.

Let's deepen your understanding of how to manage and treat each type of skin according to Ayurveda.

Vata Skin Treatment & Maintenance - First and foremost, living a *vata* balancing lifestyle and consuming a *vata* pacifying diet is critical when looking at the health of your skin. In addition, the *vata* skin-type needs proper hydration and nourishment in order to stay lively and vibrant. The consumption of warm water, warmed cow's or goat's milk is also great for the nourishment of your skin. The proper cleansing of your skin is critical in that you do not want to use harsh or drying skin applications. Doing so will only further increase the space and air elements of the *vata dosha*. Also, the consumption of healthy fats is a blessing for this dryer and thinner skin-type. And no, this does not mean bacon!

Pitta Skin Treatment & Maintenance - By being of medium thickness, the *pitta* skin-type is more prone to rashes, acne, and sores when experiencing an imbalance. Being aware of it's over sensitive nature due to the fact that it can suffer oftentimes from inflammation, is the main factor when looking to care for and treat this skin-type. Consuming foods of a cooling nature, as well as avoiding excess exposure to heat and direct sunlight is crucial in taming it's fiery nature. As mentioned before, avoiding prolonged emotional states of anger and jealousy (only to name a few) is an important aspect when looking at the "inside / out" care of your skin. Lastly, aloe it up and shower yourself in rose!

Kapha Skin Treatment & Maintenance - Enhancing this skin-types natural blessings is not always a blessing in and of itself. By being the thickest of all the skin-types, the skin of the *kapha* type is easily prone to blackheads due to its overly oily nature. The pores appear larger than most other skin types, and the retention of excess water is a concern you need to be aware of. Let me ask you, does it make sense to moisturize this skin-type within the same manner and frequency of the others? Given *kapha* skin's proclivity to overproduce oiliness, applications consisting of turmeric and clary sage are helpful to maintain the skin's natural sebum balance. In terms of a carrier oils, grapeseed oil tends to be the best choice for this skin-type due to the fact that it is lightweight yet still has sufficient amounts of omega-6, antioxidants, and linoleic acid, all of which fight the inflammation associated with acne-prone skin.

Skin Care, the Outside In Approach

You must ask yourself, how does my skin respond in certain situations and what are the more typical manifestation you experience? Are you prone to inflammation, dryness or excessive moisture and oiliness? Or perhaps your skin has always been sensitive, either to certain climatic conditions or certain foods. These I can tell you with certainly are not to be viewed as minor nuisances nor should they be chalked up to "that's just how I am". They are your body's way, or even more specific, your skin's way of letting you know something is out of whack and needs your immediate attention. From Ayurveda's perspective, most imbalances do not steam from superficial factors, meaning external factors affecting the overall health of your skin. The maintenance of your skin is a very unique balance of an emotional-physical ecology that lies within the gross and subtle levels of being. The usual root causes of skin-related disorders usually can be found residing in the following:

- the digestive system
- the blood
- the liver
- any imbalances in vata, pitta, and kapha
- emotional disturbances

- the season

This does not mean, however, that topically treating and managing your skin should be ignored or not utilized - it most certainly should. With that said, let us look at some common *doshic* related topical applications in the maintenance and treatment of your unique skin-type.

Self-massage, or as you've already learned, *abhyanga*, is one of the most effective modalities when looking to treat the skin topically. The process of self-massage calms and lubricates the skin, penetrates and cleanses the sweat glands, settles the nervous system, helps to hydrate and rejuvenate all of the tissues, and promotes healthy circulation[74]. In the morning, before a shower or bath, massage about ¼ cup of oil into the skin, of course, you'll want to use oils which are pacifying to your unique *dosha and* skin-type. Oil-based massages are particularly good at pacifying sensitive or reactive skin and can help to soothe the skin after a sunburn.

If you or your skin fosters the nature of the *kapha dosha*, then performing a dry rub is highly recommended by this author. A base of chickpea or almond flower and various paste-like applications have been used to stimulate the lymphatic system. This gets things moving, so to speak, which encourages detoxification. This slightly different version of *abhyanga* is excellent for *kapha* and *pitta doshas*. I would avoid if you're prone to sensitive skin. By

---

[74] Lad, Vasant. Textbook of Ayurveda Vol III: General Principles of Management and Treatment. Albuquerque: The Ayurvedic Press, 2012. Print. 116-118.

increasing circulation, it stimulates the liquefying of fat and helps to remove excess oil from the skin[75]. A powder can be used in conjunction with or instead of a more traditional oil massage, depending on your constitution, your current state of balance and seasonality. Chickpea is often used due to it producing a drying effect. It is astringent in taste and is an excellent skin scrubber. This practice can be performed daily or as needed. We can take a deeper look together later in your customized version.

Finally, let's take a second here and talk about soaps and the use of soap on the skin. Ayurveda does not suggest the daily use of detergent and chemically scented soap as a safe and effective option for skin management. They produce excessive dryness and are harsh. The *vata* type of skin needs to avoid or use caution here. I recommend using soaps sparingly and soap that contains oils such as neem. Neem is one of the best oils to use in the health and management of the skin, especially for *pitta* skin-types due to its cooling and soothing nature. The process of *abhyanga* followed immediately by a warm bath or shower is more than effective in the cleaning of the skin, as well as offering exfoliation. Your skin will thank you...

Protecting the Skin From Harm

Your skin is unique and so often misunderstood. Being the largest organ of the human body and one of our natural lines of defense from external harm,

---

[75] Welch, Claudia. Dinacharya: Changing Lives Through Daily Living. 2007. PDF File. 13. Online Version of Article.

the protection of your skin is something that should never be overlooked or taken for granted.

According to Ayurveda, *pitta* is responsible for the color, texture, and temperature of our skin, as well as its luster and glow. It governs the function of sweating, processes everything that we apply externally to the skin (lotions, soaps, medications, oils, etc.) and digests anything that contacts the skin more passively like dust, chemicals, irritants, and allergens[76]. Being a main seat for *pitta* in the body, the governing and balancing of this particular *dosha* is crucial in the protection of your skin - even if you're predominance does not reside in the *pitta dosha*. Now, this is not to say that avoidance or ignorance towards the other two body-types should be exercised. Who you are and how you arrived at this particular point in your life is more important than any one imbalance. This becomes especially true when looking to protect your skin.

The main protective measure under the realm of Ayurveda I just spoke of above, however, there are several other factors you need to be aware of when looking to protect the outer layer of your body. Here is a condensed list:

- Avoiding or reducing prolonged exposure to sun, especially *pitta's*
- Avoid artificial tanning - this is true for all body & skin types
- Avoidance of excessive beautification, yes there such as thing as too much

---

[76] Lad, Vasant. Textbook of Ayurveda Vol I: Fundamental Principles of Ayurveda. Albuquerque: The Ayurvedic Press, 2002. Print. 55, 64-65.

- Avoidance of over the counter beauty products containing chemical, petroleum and plastic-based derivatives
- Proper balancing of hormones offers increased skin health, protection and durability
- Proper daily self-massaging; the application of *doshic* specific oils offers added levels of skin protection
- Proper protection from extreme climatic conditions; bitter cold weather for *kapha*, extreme dry climates for *vata*, and hot and humid conditions for *pitta*

The above may seem somewhat basic, however, some of the more basic aspects of life can either produce the most harmful or most beneficial results. Can you see how the above suggestions relates directly to your daily routine?

Hair Care

The length, look, texture and color of our hair has been a focal point for men and women alike for longer than I can begin to imagine. Being more of an emphasis than even our skin and second to the appearance of our face, our hair has occupied a majority of the beauty industry since its conception. Hair, as you can possibly fathom, is more than its length, style and color. Like the health and treatment of our skin, Ayurveda's take on the maintenance and health of one's hair is fully in line with its overall premise and philosophical foundation.

Like the slew of harmful chemical additions to our skin care products, the more popular hair care products of today are no different. Seeing that the skin of the scalp is far more susceptible to becoming clogged than most other areas of the epidermis found throughout the human body, the safety of what we apply to our head and scalp becomes something which we all need to be concerned and aware of when looking at external applications. Not only do the majority of mainstream hair care products contain potentially harmful ingredients, they're damaging to the hair and superficially or temporarily treat the hair. The goal of this chapter is to introduce you to a system of beautification that can sustain and promote a sense of balance, as well as educate you on aspects of the health industry where most Americans are ignorant at best.

Sticking within the intrinsic aspects of holism, Ayurveda takes a unique approach towards the health and beautification of your hair - address the root cause, uncover your *dosha* and its current state and employ naturally occurring compounds of a therapeutic and opposite nature. Relating the state of your digestion (*agni*) to the health of your hair is a concept here in the West that was lost, or perhaps, never fully adopted. This leads us down a path where your diet, state of digestion and your overall mental health becomes the source for the health and vibrancy of your hair. My goal in writing this section of this book is designed to not only educate you on these unique applications and their hard to pronounce words, but bring forth a systematic set of tools that you can use in place of or in conjunction with your current health and beauty practices. Despite common conjecture, Ayurveda offers a number of impressive beautification strategies that are easy, safe and produce long lasting results. Let's take a look at these strategies in relation to the health and vibrancy of your hair.

Your skin and hair alike fall under the same *doshic* principles as does every other aspect of your mental and physical being. So, yes, there is a *vata* hair-type, a *pitta* hair-type and a *kapha* hair-type. Your unique bodily constitution and its current state directly relates to the health and appearance of your hair. Allow me to take a few moments to share with you the three hair-types and their unique characteristics as brought forth by Ayurveda.

Vata Hair-Type - The *vata* hair-type is the thinnest of all the types, and can often described as course. It grows quickly, and if not properly managed, can become a bit unruly making it harder to style.

Common *vata* imbalance of the hair manifests as hair that's dry and frizzy. If your hair seems to lack luster this will point you towards an imbalance of *vata dosha*. Hair featuring ends that break and split easily, as well as clumps of hair falling out is a strong indicator of an imbalance within this constitution. When in balance, the *vata* hair-type will grow quickly, however, when it is suffering from a disorder stemming from a vitiation of the *vata dosha*, it will grow very slowly and come in thin.

Pitta Hair-Type - The *pitta* hair-type is is straight, soft, predictable and of moderate thickness. It can tend to be on the fine side and often times can turn gray more rapidly than the other *doshas*.

Common *pitta* imbalances of the hair can cause excess heat within the hair follicles and damage the hair, leading to premature thinning, early greying, and baldness. Heat in the hair follicles is often accompanied by a tendency to be hot-headed, short- tempered or excessively ambitious. The importance here to understand is that imbalances do not only manifest within the physical realm, they can manifest and be diagnosed under the seat of mental imbalances as well.

Kapha Hair-Type - The *kapha* hair-type is typically wavy, lustrous, full, strong, coarse, and thick. This look is often the most sought after, however, it certainly does not mean its the best - that is purely subjective.

Common *kapha* imbalances relating to your hair can be witnessed as an excessive oiliness, heaviness and thickness of the hair. The appearance of hair suffering from an imbalance of this nature will be heavy and flat. Excessive shampooing will not only offer any relief from the imbalance itself, but will further damage the hair strands and follicles. At this point the only remedy after the *doshic* imbalance is corrected is to cut off the dead hair. The good news...it will grow back full and thick.

If you believe your hair is not healthy then the first course of action is to discover the type of hair you have, assuming that you've already assessed your specific *dosha*. It is magnificent that all diagnostic procedures under the realm of Ayurveda are the same throughout the entire scope of this beautiful system of healthcare. One aspect that you must understand, and perhaps may not fully be in line with yet, is that you need to flow with the natural rhythms of your body (and your hair-type in this instance). The results will not only be the most successful, but they're the safest and will produce long lasting results. I bring this up because the standard today seemingly tends to lean toward the *kapha* hair-type as the gold standard for all. This is not only purely subjective, but can lead you towards unsafe and damaging practices. Like I said in the very beginning of this work, understand who you truly are and celebrate and enhance the flow of your true nature. Remember, you can only move forward upstream for so long before it knocks you down and you begin to flow backwards.

The Mind, Stress & Your Hair

Most disorders relating to the hair often stem from an imbalance of the *vata dosha*. If chronic stress is a common disorder that can be directly related to the *vata dosha*, then it stands to reason that managing your daily stressors can be vital to the look and health of your hair. When you perceive a threat the body activates the fight or flight response, thus releasing a plethora of stress-related hormones such as adrenaline and cortisol. The problem here lies in the fact that most of our daily stresses are non-life threatening, however, your nervous system cannot tell the difference. Arguing with your kids over doing their homework in a timely manner, cramming for a work deadline or being chased by a blood hungry bear activates the release of the same hormones. The only difference being that if you were to escape the grips of the hungry bear your physio-emotional state will return to a state of homeostasis as soon as the threat is removed. The constant emotional triggers we as humans choose to deal with day in and day out keeps us on a constant state of alert, thus forcing the continual release of stress hormones. By residing under a constant state of stress a vitiation of the *vata dosha* (possibly one of the others as well) is sure to follow. Not only does residing in a continued state of stress cause an imbalance of the *doshas*, it also robs your organs and tissues of critical nutrients its needs for growth. Your hair, if you don't already know, is made of proteins filaments, or keratin. While residing in a state of stress, as you learned from the chapter "[Digestion, Do You Get it?]()," greatly affects your state of digestion. When your digestive state is not working effectively the digestion and assimilation of the food substances such as fats and proteins becomes hampered. This directly affects the health of your hair. The process is quite simple...

The Inside Out Approach to Hair Health

The entire approach to Ayurveda stems from degeneration and regeneration. It's approach to the health and growth of your hair is no different. The proper nourishment of bodily organs and tissues (hair follicles) via a robust state of digestion breeds growth and cellular production. When looking at an internal approach to the health of your hair, just as in the health of your skin, the state of your digestion becomes one of the most critical aspects to the health of your hair and skin. Oh, and do not forget, to consume healthy and *dosha* specific foods. When that is not enough, there are other avenues of treatment you can employ to help you realize your fullest endeavors when wearing a beautiful head of hair. Under the umbrella of the Ayurvedic traditions, there is a section on rejuvenation, called *rasayana* in Sanskrit[77]. Rejuvenation through proper nourishment affects the body at a cellular and energetic levels, hence helping to control the growth, luster and overall health of your hair. There are numerous herbal and mineral-based remedies that have been used for centuries in the treatment of hair. The amazing thing here, is that the herbs suggested by Ayurveda for the fullness, luster, growth and health of your hair has its efficacy in cellular rejuvenation, thus when looking to promote healthy hair you are in fact aiding in the rejuvenation of all of your bodily tissues and organs. This directly relates back to the law of cause and effect.

There are many wonderful herbs and herbal compounds that have a positive effect on the health of your hair. I am surely not going to list them all, but will certainly reference a few that have been known to produce excellent results in the growth and treatment of your hair when consumed orally. As you'll read in the coming section, most of these herbs can be transitioned and used topically as well.

---

[77] "Rasayana - Wikipedia." https://en.wikipedia.org/wiki/Rasayana. Accessed 9 June. 2018.

Amalaki - Amalaki is one of the three ingredients used in *triphala*. Used as a singular compound, it offers potent rejuvenation properties, as well as being a potent antioxidant. By being cool in nature, it is a go to herb for subsiding the increased heat of the fire element, thus helping to cool and strengthen the hair follicles.

Triphala - Yes, again with the three flowers! *Triphala* is a powerhouse when it comes to detoxification and rejuvenation, so needless to say, it has been used for the treatment of health hair for many generations. It's true efficacy in the treatment of your hair lies in its potent digestive building properties. As you just learned, digestion is not only the key to the health of your hair but to your entire mind and body.

Bhringaraj - Yea, this is a toughie to pronounce, nevertheless, it has been referred to as the ruler of the hair! It's strong affinity towards the health of your hair follicles makes this one of the most powerful herbs when looking at the growth and regeneration of your hair. This wonder herb is for the most part balancing in moderation for all three *doshas*, however, it does possess more of a cooling nature. By being slightly cooling it is very effective in taming the excess *pitta*, thus, making it very effective in the treatment of hair loss, luster and battling the oftentimes unwanted greys!

The Outside In Approach to Hair Health

I am a firm believer that true beauty comes from within, however, with that said, there are several effective topical applications and treatments used under the scope of Ayurveda that I want to share with you. Treating your hair and scalp directly can offer many health and beauty benefits. Unbeknownst to most, the skin of the scalp is quite thick, though it contains many more follicles than the rest of the body. Given this fact, the scalp has a greater tendency to become dirtier, so to speak, than most other areas of epidermis covering the body. You sweat a lot more via the scalp than you're probably aware of, thus increasing the likelihood of clogged hair follicles. Combine the sweat and dirt with chemical residue, and you are setting the health of your scalp and hair up for disaster.

One benefit of topically treating and maintaining your hair is that you do not need to be suffering from an imbalance in order to prosper from its many applications. Improving the health and look of your hair can be performed easily and effectively through this system of care.

Direct scalp applications or superficial applications of certain herbal formulas applied directly to your scalp can offer a host of health benefits. Like the rest of your skin, your scalp has the ability to absorb nutrients directly. This as you can imagine, it is a double-sided sword; it will absorb unhealthy things just as easily as healthy things.

Another very beneficial aspect of topical applications is the fact that when nutritive formulas are applied directly to the scalp they get carried through the physical and energetic channels of the body. By utilizing the correct oil-based carrier, the influence can be wide-spread, thus producing positive effects. In addition, the scalp offers direct access to the subtler aspects of the mind, or as it is referred to in Sanskrit, *marmas*[78]. An application of the proper oil-based remedy directly to the scalp not only moisturizes and strengthens the strands of your hair, but it nourishes the cells, stimulates the flow of blood which promotes regeneration and growth. Now, you cannot merely apply random oils and herbs to your scalp. Remember, even this needs to be *doshic* and imbalance specific. With that said, here are a few unique hair treatment applications for each of the *tridoshas*.

Vata Hair Treatment - In a small bowl make a paste consisting of 3oz. sesame oil with ⅓ cup of *triphala* powder. Let the combination infuse for several hours. Part the hair, thus exposing the scalp. With your index and middle fingers, apply the oil directly to the scalp. Repeat in an adjacent area of the scalp and repeat again until the full scalp is covered. In a circular motion massage the scalp. This stimulates the flow of blood to the scalp. Let it sit for an hour or so and then wash off with an organic-based, non-harsh shampoo. Warm water alone can be sufficient enough.

---

[78] "Do this Marma Point Scalp Massage with Newly Discovered ...." 19 Jan. 2017, https://lifespa.com/marma-point-scalp-massage-newly-discovered-benefits/. Accessed 11 June. 2018.

The heating action of the sesame oil, combined with the balancing and rejuvenating effects of *triphala* powder produces a powerful *vata* balancing mask for your scalp and hair.

Pitta Hair Treatment - In a small bowl make a paste consisting of 3oz. of organic, raw and plain yogurt with ⅓ cup of amalaki powder. Let the combination infuse for several hours. Part the hair, exposing the scalp. Repeat in an adjacent area of the scalp and repeat again until the full scalp is covered. In a circular motion massage the scalp, thus stimulating the flow of blood. Let the infusion absorb for an hour plus and then wash off with an organic-based, non-harsh shampoo of a cooling nature (neem-based shampoo is a wise choice).

Since yogurt is rich in the water and earth elements it produces a pacifying effect for the *pitta dosha*. Combined with the cooling energetics of amalaki, this becomes a very potent hair and scalp mask in the treatment of premature balding and greying of the hair.

Kapha Hair Treatment - In a small bowl make a paste consisting 3oz. of olive oil and mustard seed oil, blended with with ⅓ cup of *triphala* powder. Let the combination infuse for several hours. Part the hair, exposing the scalp and apply the infusion directly onto the scalp. Continue to repeat in adjacent areas of the scalp until the full scalp is covered. In a circular motion, massage the scalp, thereby stimulating the flow of blood. Let the oily sit for an hour and then wash with an organic-based shampoo. A more aggressive shampoo can be used here due to the naturally oily nature of the *kapha* hair.

Typically, of the all the hair-types, *kapha* hair needs the least maintenance. This, of course, is not always the case and this is not a prescription to avoid performing proper hair maintenance. The excess of *kapha* makes the scalp more vulnerable to the accumulation of excess dirt, thus clogging the pores and making your scalp more prone to infections and or dandruff. Given the often oily nature of the *kapha* type hair, more frequent washing is advised.

Protecting the Hair From Harm

Protection or preventative procedures are always the best line of defense when it comes to the health of any aspect or area of the body. Your hair is certainly no exception to this rule. Typically one's hair is often more abused than most surface aspects of the body. There are several common practices that are damaging to your hair. Some are obvious, like burning via a flat iron, but some are less obvious. Here is a list of the more common harmful hair practices that you should avoid or greatly reduce:

- Excessive ironing or overheating the hair via blow drying
- Excessive showering with hot water
- Excessive washing
- Bleaching
- Chlorine, via pools and hot tubs

- Chemical-based hair dyes
- Abrasive and chemically laden shampoos and other various hair care products

I am not saying you should fully avoid the practices listed above, whereas anything in light moderation will not under normal circumstances have any profound negative effects. What you need to be aware of, however, is that even one application of hair bleaching can greatly damage your hair. There are several remedies that you can use in order to limit the adverse effects of hair bleaching and coloring. The first and foremost is to make sure the health of your hair is in an optimal state. Hair that is weak or is currently suffering from an imbalance will not be able to recover from even one session of bleaching or chemically treated coloring. Proper hydration of the hair strands can offer protective aspects when it comes to bleaching and hair coloring.

Once you fully accept, learn and incorporate the importance of your daily routine, only then will you become the master and no longer fall victim to being the servant to superficial and external experiences. Take a single step each day towards wellness, prosperity and happiness and build upon that positivity each day moving forward. The formation of your daily habits that are built upon the foundational aspects of this book will unconsciously guide you towards living the life you once could only see in your deepest reverie.

Summation

"Ayurveda teaches us to cherish our innate-nature – "to love and honor who we are", not as what people think or tell us, "who we should be."

- Prana Gogia

As you've discovered within the many pages of this book, Ayurveda is more than a system for treating disease - it is a way of life. Despite its origins dating back over 5,000 years ago, its foundation is still valid and alive today. It has taught us that there is an energetic undercurrent connecting all things, all the time and in all places. It guides you towards a deeper understanding of how we as humans are related and are undeniably connected to the basic elements of life - elements of which comprise all living and nonliving things. Following this premise, the importance of consuming foods that were created by the air, sun, water and earth should now be the foundation of your life moving forward. By consuming a diet consisting of fresh organic foods, you are in turn ingesting the living and energetic aspects of the universal elements. Can you fathom a simpler concept - build our medicines right into our food?

At the core of this ancient science is you; your unique collection of the physical, mental and spiritual characteristics stemming from the 5 basic elements of the universe. By educating and guiding you through the days, seasons and stages of life, the main goal of this system of health is to keep you free from disease and to assist you in living a life full of happiness and love - what better gift!

Having provided us the wisdom in understanding the constant fluctuations of life, Ayurveda has also passed down easy, safe and effective remedies for those particular times in your life when you drift away from your God-given tendencies. These timeless therapies consider you as a whole entity and from here a systematic process has been brought forth in returning you to a balanced state. You see, residing within a cooperative union with the natural rhythms of the universe is your mind and body's unconscious goal, despite the fact that it has been lost and forgotten by the egoic nature of our conscious minds. In essense, you are not learning something new, but rather remembering something forgotten - something that is innate within all humans regardless of age, sex, religious beliefs or creed. We are all one with one common goal - it's simply that most of us have forgotten and have lost our way.

The methodologies provided within the many pages of this book is a system that anyone can use anywhere, at anytime and during any stage of life. The true wisdom and magic of Ayurveda melds with your true nature - it doesn't fight it. The goal in writing this book for you was to educate, enlighten and guide you out of the darkness of sickness and disease and into the light of living a life full of true health and true happiness. I have seen first hand the beauty and simplistic nature of this science provide miracles for many who had nowhere else to turn. My question to you is why wait! Needing to hit rock bottom in order to begin to change is another one of the many falsehoods created by the greed of the few. Are you ready to break free from the standard of care in this country; keep 'em sick and keep 'em coming back?

If the honest answer to this question is yes, then do not worry for you're now holding the key to unlock the shackles of greed and corruption at the highest level. Read, digest and adopt the practices provided within and change will happen as sure as the sun will set tonight to only rise yet again tomorrow.

If you the information found within this book is not able to help you achieve all of your health and wellness endeavors, than it would be my pleasure in further helping reach your specific goals. Remember, without knowing your unique body-type, its current state and the set of specific challenges you face, I cannot offer anything other than what I've provided in this work.

My door is open and waiting for your correspondence - Namaste!

Scott Blaise

Letter From the Editor

Scottie is a hottie in ma bottie, waiting on JA-JA-JA JEWLY!

www.ingramcontent.com/pod-product-compliance
Lightning Source LLC
Chambersburg PA
CBHW060825220526
45466CB00003B/977